ANTIRACISM NURSING AND MIDWIFERY

Many nurses and midwives, qualified or in training, and their patients, experience racism in the healthcare system. This change-oriented book, based on the knowledge and experiences of people who have lived experience of being Black and minoritised bodies within the professions, and scholars who write and research on the topics, seeks to challenge the status quo.

Exploring the Western centrism of contemporary healthcare and education that contributes to racialised and health disparities, this innovative ground-breaking book explores the historical and theoretical context of racism in contemporary nursing and midwifery. It goes on to look at the contribution that leadership and education can make to antiracism changes in practice. There are specific topics in chapters discussing whistle-blowing, the impact of covid, the experiences of international nurses and a case study of Welsh nursing antiracism policy. Each chapter takes a pragmatic approach, looking at how to implement antiracism change, ending with a reflection activity for the reader to complete. Intending to mobilise the profession to engage in antiracism policy, practice and education strategically and collaboratively for an equitable and just way of being and doing nursing and midwifery.

This book is an important read for nursing and midwifery students, professionals, educators and leaders.

Musharrat J. Ahmed-Landeryou is Associate Professor and Professional Lead in Occupational Therapy at London South Bank University, where she leads the School of Allied and Community Health's decolonising strategy.

"This book is a courageous and insightful examination of racism in nursing and midwifery, revealing how inequality persists despite decades of policy driven solutions. Through the combined power of Critical Race Theory and studies it exposed the hidden dynamics woven into systems, cultures and everyday practice. Using real life case studies, it brings to light the structural forces that undermine fairness and compromise the wellbeing of both staff and patients. This work challenges readers to confront uncomfortable truths while offering a clear pathway to meaningful reform. Personally, I believe this is essential reading for all who are committed to creating a just, compassionate and inclusive profession."

Michelle Cox, *FRCN FQICN, Michelle Cox Consultancy*

"This book takes the reader on a rigorous and critically informed journey that positions antiracism as foundational to nursing and midwifery theory and practice. Drawing on Critical Race Theory, it makes visible the structural, institutional, and everyday manifestations of racism within the professions, offering clear definitions alongside grounded examples. Interwoven throughout the chapters are emancipatory concepts and practices that invite the reader into acts of critical reflection and praxis. In doing so, the book moves beyond description to action, equipping nurses and midwives to challenge inequity, advance justice, and support care practices that recognise and uphold the value of all life. It is essential reading not only for practitioners, but also for policy makers, managers and leaders, whose decisions shape education, workforce cultures, and health systems, providing critical insights to inform equitable policy, ethical leadership, and systemic change."

Professor Joy Warmington, *CEO BRAP (Birmingham Race Action Partnership)*

"This book is important and transformative. The book is a powerful and necessary examination of racism and antiracism in nursing and midwifery. Combining scholarship with lived experience, it supports professionals, leaders, policy makers and students to critically reflect on practice, confront structural inequities, and commit to actions, creating more socially just, inclusive, and compassionate nursing and midwifery to change the status quo."

Professor Gina Awoko Higginbottom, *MBE, FQICN, FAAN*
Emeritus Professor of Ethnicity and Community Health, School of Health Sciences, University of Nottingham, Adjunct Professor, University of Alberta, Canada

ANTIRACISM NURSING AND MIDWIFERY

From Praxis to Action

Edited by Musharrat J. Ahmed-Landeryou

Routledge
Taylor & Francis Group
LONDON AND NEW YORK

Designed cover image: Getty

First published 2027
by Routledge
4 Park Square, Milton Park, Abingdon, Oxon OX14 4RN

and by Routledge
605 Third Avenue, New York, NY 10158

Routledge is an imprint of the Taylor & Francis Group, an informa business

British Library Cataloguing-in-Publication Data
A catalogue record for this book is available from the British Library

Library of Congress Cataloging-in-Publication Data
Names: Ahmed-Landeryou, Musharrat J. editor
Title: Anti-racism nursing and midwifery : from praxis to action /
[edited by Musharrat J. Ahmed-Landeryou].
Description: Abingdon, Oxon ; New York, NY : Routledge, 2026. |
Includes bibliographical references and index. |
Identifiers: LCCN 2026009078 (print) | LCCN 2026009079 (ebook) |
ISBN 9781032933184 hbk | ISBN 9781032933177 pbk | ISBN 9781003565369 ebk
Subjects: LCSH: Nursing--Social aspects | Midwifery--Social aspects |
Racism in medicine--Prevention | Anti-racism in medicine |
Discrimination in medical care--Prevention | Race
Classification: LCC RT86.5 .A57 2026 (print) | LCC RT86.5 (ebook)
LC record available at https://lccn.loc.gov/2026009078
LC ebook record available at https://lccn.loc.gov/2026009079

ISBN: 978-1-032-93318-4 (hbk)
ISBN: 978-1-032-93317-7 (pbk)
ISBN: 978-1-003-56536-9 (ebk)

DOI: 10.4324/9781003565369

Typeset in Times New Roman
by KnowledgeWorks Global Ltd.

CONTENTS

ABOUT THE EDITOR

Musharrat J. Ahmed-Landeryou, PhD, is Associate Professor and Professional Lead in Occupational Therapy at London South Bank University, where she leads the School of Allied and Community Health's decolonising strategy. Her decolonising the curriculum wheel is part of her university's curriculum quality framework. Also, she co-founded BAMEOTUK, a network of Black and minoritised occupational therapy students, staff and educators working to address institutional racism in the profession and its education. She delivers workshops for antiracism or decolonising for curriculum/higher education/organisational change. She is a history maker in occupational therapy by sole editing the book "Anti-racist Occupational Therapy: Unsettling the status quo" a topic not raised in the profession's literature till then.

CONTRIBUTORS

Precious Adade Duodu, PhD, is a Senior Lecturer in Adult Nursing and the International Lead in Nursing at the University of Huddersfield, UK. A thought leader in nursing education, regulation and workforce development, he co-chairs his University's Black Staff Affinity Group and serves as a Member of the Chief Nursing Officer's and Chief Midwifery Officer's Black and Minority Ethnic Strategic Advisory Group (NHS England), shaping inclusive policy and championing race equality in higher education and healthcare. He has been instrumental in strengthening nursing and midwifery regulation in Ghana, being instrumental in the introduction of the national revalidation policy for nurses and midwives (the first ever in an LMIC). Also, he has led impactful projects addressing non-communicable diseases (NCDs), particularly diabetes and dementia in Ghana and serves as co-investigator for NCD projects in other LMICs (India and Nepal). With over a decade of global experience, he advances anti-racist education, health equity and capacity building across the UK and LMICs to shape inclusive and socially just nursing practice globally. Internationally, he serves as a Visiting Senior Lecturer at the Kwame Nkrumah University of Science and Technology (KNUST), Ghana. He is a Fellow of both Advance HE (FHEA) and the Royal Society for Public Health (FRSPH).

Yetunde Akinnuoye, is Senior Lecturer and Programme Director for the Master's programme at City University of London, as well as the Lead for the Learning and Teaching Committee. She brings a strong clinical background in midwifery with extensive expertise in the high-risk management of pregnancy. Her academic work includes conducting an empirical review of North Central London's *Better Births: Improving Care in the Community for Vulnerable Women*, which critically examines the challenges and opportunities within midwifery care for vulnerable populations. Additionally, she has contributed to the Twinning Project, coordinated by the Royal College of Midwives, which underscores the importance of academic support in advancing pedagogical practices within midwifery education. She is deeply committed to advancing both the practical and pedagogical aspects of midwifery education, ensuring that both academic frameworks and clinical practices are aligned to meet the needs of diverse and vulnerable populations.

Shadrach Dare, PhD, is a registered Nurse from Ghana and a member of the UK Faculty for Public Health. He is currently a Lecturer in Nursing and Public Health at Glasgow Caledonian University where he co-leads the Public Health programme. Dr Dare has wide Nursing and Public Health experiences across Africa, Europe and America. His research interests span across maternal and child health, education and inequalities where he applies quantitative and mixed methods research approaches to understanding and promoting health among disadvantaged communities. Shadrach is also passionate about EDI which is reflected in his teaching and student supervision.

Linda Deravin (Professor), RN, PhD, MHM, GCert LTHE, GCert ARRN, GDip Ger, GCert E Health, BN, is a proud Wiradjuri woman and is the Head of School and Dean for the School of Nursing and Midwifery at the University of Southern Queensland, Australia. Throughout her nursing career she has worked as a clinician, educator and both an executive nurse and a health manager in a variety of settings. Linda continues to work with a variety of communities to pursue her research interests in First Nations health and education, aged care, chronic care and health workforce issues.

Richard Desir, MA, BSc (Hons), DipN, DMS, PgCert, RN, is a Nursing Officer in the office of the Chief Nursing Officer, Welsh Government, leading on patient experience and NHS safeguarding. He champions inclusive healthcare policy and practice, contributing to national antiracism initiatives and supporting underrepresented voices in nursing and midwifery. Richard is dedicated to embedding equity, diversity and inclusion across the NHS, ensuring patient experiences drive meaningful change.

Michelle Dillon, EdD, PhD, is a Senior Lecturer in nurse education with extensive experience across both clinical and academic settings. She began her career in the NHS in 1999 as a children's cancer nurse, before moving into full-time higher education in 2013. Michelle completed her Professional Doctorate in 2025 at the University of Bath. Her thesis, "The international nurse: culture and communication in the NHS," explored the complex dynamics of cultural identity, communication and professional integration and crucially, highlighted the persistent racism and discrimination faced by internationally educated nurses and UK-born Black and minoritised healthcare workers. As a White ally, Michelle actively uses her academic platform to amplify minoritised and marginalised voices, challenge systemic inequities and promote anti-racist practice in healthcare education.

Anton Emmanuel (Professor), is a Physician and Researcher since 1990, who has worked in inclusion and leadership in national organisations since the start of the COVID-19 pandemic. The intention in the inclusion space has been to mirror the clinical. Namely to use data to identify the specific problems where targeted change is needed, allied to then implementing evidence-based actions that transform those problems. Working currently with the Welsh Government is beginning to transfer this theory of change into practice.

Sarah Esegbona-Adeigbe, PhD, RM, RGN, Associate Professor Midwifery, London South Bank University, is the Course Leader for the postgraduate diploma in midwifery at London South Bank University and has specialist knowledge and experience in complications in pregnancy, cultural safety, cultural competency, haemoglobinopathies, female genital mutilation and racial disparities in maternal and women's health. Sarah contributed extensively to decolonising the midwifery curriculum at London South Bank University and continues to do equality, diversity and inclusion (EDI) work to improve students' experiences. Sarah recently completed her PhD exploring migrant Nigerian mothers' and midwives' perceptions of cultural competency in antenatal care. Her book "Transcultural Midwifery Practice" addressed a gap in the literature that equipped midwifery students and midwives to cater for diverse childbearing populations.

Nathalya Fonseca Camargo, Midwife, Master's student, Midwife graduated from the University of São Paulo (USP), Public Health Specialist and Master in Public Health from the USP School of Public Health, with an emphasis on obstetric racism and the comprehensive health of the Black population. She works at Fiocruz/Ministry of Health in the project Strategy to Confront Racism in Health and is a member of the research group Gender, Motherhood, and Health (GEMAS). Founder of Maoni – Gestar e Nascer, where she develops actions in gynaecological and obstetric care, female self-care, as well as lectures and training on the health of the Black population.

Vanessa Heaslip (Professor) PhD, MA, BSc (Hons), DipHE, RN, DN, is a Professor of Nursing and Healthcare Equity at Salford University. Her research interests are in communities who experience health inequity and social exclusion and whose voices are not traditionally heard in the academic and professional discourse. She has worked with a variety of groups including Gypsy, Roma, Travellers, people living with mental health issues, people in prison and people from ethnic and racialised communities. In recognition for her work, Professor Heaslip has received numerous awards including Sigma International Nurse Researcher Hall of Fame (2025), Chief Nurse Award for Adult Social Care (2025), Royal College of Nursing

Northwest Award for Outstanding Contribution to Equality, Diversity and Inclusion (2024), Burdett Hero Award (2022) and Woman of the Year (2019).

Mushtag Kahin is registered Nursing Associate and current MSc Mental Health Nursing Student. She is a graduate of the MSc in Mental Health Studies and works as a part-time Project Lead. She has previous NHS experience as a mental health practitioner and management of Link Workers, Duty in a community mental health team and crisis resolution home treatment team. Mushtag is passionate about transcultural leadership and anti-racist leadership in the NHS.

Hal King, MRES, BA, is an advocacy caseworker at the charity Friends, Families and Travellers, a national organisation that provides support to Gypsy, Roma and Traveller communities. With a Master of Research degree in philosophy, Hal is continuing his academic career as an independent scholar, with research interest in environmental philosophy, as well as decolonisation. On the interface between research and advocacy, his charity work is complemented by academic research, applying praxis informed by ethical theory. Driven by the values of social and environmental justice, Hal was drawn to the work that FFT does to uphold the nomadic way of life, allowing for intimate relationships with the natural world and one's environment to blossom freely.

Miranda Leach, RM, BSc, MSc, PGCE, SFHEA, is a Senior Midwifery Lecturer at the School of Health & Medical Sciences, City St George's, University of London, and also a previous fellow of Council of Deans of Health. I have over 20 years of clinical experience and came into teaching in 2016. I have a passion for advocating for women, the under privileged and vulnerable. I am equally committed to ensuring midwifery students are equipped with the necessary knowledge and skills at the point of registration to provide evidence-based, compassionate, women-centred holistic care. I am currently undergoing my doctoral studies at the University College London.

Patricia Lima Ferreira Santa Rosa (Professor), RN, Midwife, PhD, Nurse Midwife, Associate Professor at the Ribeirão Preto College of Nursing, University of São Paulo (EERP-USP). She earned her PhD (2018) and MSc (2013) in Nursing Science from the University of São Paulo School of Nursing (EEUSP), RN – Obstetric Nursing (2010) and BSc in Nursing (2006). She is an active member of leading national research and advocacy networks, including the Racism and Health Working Group of the Brazilian Association of Collective Health (ABRASCO), the Race.ID Research Group (USP Medical School), the Research Center in Collective Health (NUPESCO/EERP-USP), the National Articulation of Black Nurses (ANEN) and the Equity Working Group of the Brazilian Nursing Association (ABEn). Her research and professional agenda focus on racial equity in health, with emphasis on the health of the Black population, ethnic-racial relations, obstetric nursing, sexual and reproductive health, psychometrics, diversity, equity and inclusion (DEI), and the nursing workforce."

Adrienne Lipscomb, RN, Grad Cert Wiradjuri language, culture and heritage. Grad Dip MHN & Indigenous trauma and recovery practice. Lipscomb is a proud Wiradjuri and Ngemba woman and experienced mental health nurse with over 15 years working across remote, forensic and child and adolescent settings. She is a Lecturer at the University of Melbourne's School of Health Sciences and an Aboriginal Senior Therapeutic Practitioner with the Victorian Aboriginal Child and Community Agency (VACCA) Aboriginal Children's Healing Team. Adrienne holds a graduate certificate in Wiradjuri Language, Culture and Heritage, a graduate diploma in Mental Health Nursing and Indigenous Trauma and Recovery and is currently completing a Master of Indigenous Health. Adrienne brings expertise in trauma-informed, culturally responsive care across both clinical and educational environments.

Rhonda Marriott (Professor), matrilineally descended from Nyikina people of the Kimberley, AM, Nurse and Midwife, has extensive senior university leadership and translational research experience. Professor Marriott is privileged to have had a long career practicing as a nurse and a midwife, and also an extensive career as an academic. As Pro Vice Chancellor of Ngangk Yira Institute for Change at Murdoch University, Professor Marriott provides strong cultural and scientific leadership that inspires the Institute's breadth of research and advocacy work for translation into policy and practice through a System and Policy's Lens – with a view to holding systems accountable and open to calibration and change. With a vision for the sustainability of this unique Aboriginal translational research Institute, she has drawn together a passionate team of Aboriginal and non-Indigenous researcher allies who have extensive professional, community and academic networks both nationally and internationally.

Hayley Mongta, RN/RM, BNur, MMid, is a proud Gunaikurnai woman, a dual registered Nurse and Midwife and currently a Lecturer in the school of nursing and midwifery at Griffith University. She has extensive clinical and educational experience and is deeply committed to advancing culturally safe, person-centred care in nursing and midwifery.

Rafaella Pires Vieira, Midwife, Master's student, Midwife graduated from the University of São Paulo (USP), with experience in women's health. Researcher in the fields of Black population health and women's health. Master's student in Public Health at the Faculty of Medicine of the University of São Paulo (FMUSP), focusing on obstetric racism. Member of the Race ID research group on Black population health. Speaker with experience in topics related to women's health and the health of the Black population.

Naheeda Rehman is a registered Children's Nurse, Health Visitor and Senior Child Nurse Lecturer at Sheffield Hallam University. She serves as the Race and Culture Lead within the Nursing & Midwifery department and is the Academic Lead for the Minoritised Student Support Group. Naheeda is also the Lead for recruitment in the undergraduate nursing & midwifery courses and has a keen interest in widening participation initiatives and inclusive recruitment practice. Naheeda has led on initiatives promoting inclusivity and equity, including the uniform hijab project, safe space drop-ins and race equity training. She has also held workshops for staff, students and practice partners, promoting collaborative anti-racist action. A passionate advocate for EDI, she is committed to creating supportive, learning environments which enhance belonging from recruitment to employment.

Tracy Reibel (Professor), As Systems and Policy Lead at the Ngangk Yira Institute for Change, Murdoch University, Western Australia, Tracy has three decades of research and advocacy expertise devoted to maternal and infant health care systems, with the recent decade focussed on Aboriginal and Torres Strait Islander women. A non-Indigenous woman born of German, Scottish and Irish ancestry, Tracy brings a diversity of life and academic experience to her collaborations and has strong and enduring connections with Indigenous peoples across Australia and internationally which continue to inform and build her knowledge and understanding. The Ngangk Yira Institute values and promotes working together as the only solution to addressing racism in health systems, and through her allyship, Tracy leads by example in efforts to decolonise research, make health systems culturally safe and support the research sovereignty of Aboriginal and Torres Strait Islander peoples.

Ifrah Salih, EdD, Associate Head of School, works at Sheffield Hallam University and is the Associate Head of the Health and Social Care School. Ifrah has a keen interest in race equity and is the founder of the Nursing and Midwifery Minoritised (NMM) group. Ifrah has recently completed her Doctorate exploring the transition experience of ethnically minoritised student nurses into university using Critical Race Theory (CRT) as the theoretical framework. Ifrah's work around race equity has led her to work with regional and national groups and is a member of the Council of Deans (Health) EDI Strategy Group.

Natalie Stake-Doucet, RN, PhD, is a Visiting Professor at Université du Québec à Montréal (UQAM), Nurse Researcher and Educator with a focus on the social and political history of nursing. Her clinical experience includes mental health and community nursing, and she works with harm reduction organizations in Montreal, Canada.

Sue Tranka, MSc (Hons, Professor), PGDip, RN, FQNI, FRCSI, is the Chief Nursing Officer for Wales and Nurse Director of NHS Wales. She has 34 years of global experience in nursing and has spent the last 26 years working in the National Health Service. Sue trained as a midwife, registered general nurse, mental health nurse and community nurse in South Africa before joining the NHS in 1999. Sue is committed to excellence in professional practice, quality improvement & patient safety. Sue is an Honorary Visiting Professor at Cardiff University. In 2020 & 2024, she was listed among the Health Service Journal's 50 most influential people in health from a Black, Asian and minority ethnic background, and in December 2021 was awarded a fellowship of the Queen's Nursing Institute and has been convened as a Fellow of the Royal College of Surgeons Ireland Nursing and Midwifery Faculty.

Timothea T. Vo PhD, RN, CTN-B, is a tenure-track Assistant Professor in the Decker College of Nursing and Health Sciences, Division of Nursing, at Binghamton University, Vestal, NY. Vo serves as the primary clinical instructor for obstetric nursing in a Northeastern hospital, educating, overseeing and evaluating over 40 nursing students, to ensure safe delivery of culturally-concordant care for childbearing people living in the rural Finger Lakes community of Upstate New York. She is the 2024 Research Article of the Year winner, awarded by *MCN, The American Journal of Maternal/Child Nursing*, for her dissertation that explored Vietnamese women's experiences of postpartum intergenerational conflict. She is board-certified in transcultural nursing and has completed a postdoctoral research fellowship in advanced sleep and circadian rhythms at Northeastern University. Her program of research grapples with Asian-American maternal child health equity. Vo completed her PhD in nursing at the University of Connecticut, where she received rigorous training in qualitative research methodologies (primary mentor: Cheryl Beck). Additionally, she is well published and a speaker at regional, national and international spaces on various topics such as Vietnamese cultural health.

Joel Wunimasim Daanyaya is a Lecturer in Adult Nursing at the University of Cumbria. With a strong commitment to social justice in nursing practice and education, Joel leads the EDI strategy for the nursing subject group at the University of Cumbria. He co-chairs the Chief Nursing Officer (CNO) of England's Professional Strategy Working Group on Research and Innovation as part of the 10 Year Health Plan (10YHP). Joel's current doctoral work researches the lived experiences of internationally educated nurses in their transition from clinical practice to nursing academia in the UK.

FOREWORD BY PROFESSOR SINEGUGU DUMA

Antiracism Nursing and Midwifery: From Praxis to Action is more than a book – it is a manifesto for change, and a beacon of hope for the future of justice-based nursing and midwifery healthcare. This book is historic, as it is the first of its kind in nursing and midwifery, it is long overdue and vital for the profession, representing a groundbreaking contribution to the global discourse on equity and justice within nursing and midwifery. It does not treat antiracism as an abstract ideal or a distant aspiration; rather, it positions it as a moral and ethical professional imperative for an actionable foundation upon which liberatory person-centred care must be started from.

The content illuminates the enduring legacies of systemic racism that shape contemporary clinical outcomes and professional cultures worldwide. Yet, this book does not stop at critical understandings. Each chapter provides both critical insight and practical actions for disrupting/dismantling inequities towards transformation, aligning with global standards such as the World Health Organization's commitment to health equity and the International Council of Nurses' emphasis on social justice. Drawing on interdisciplinary frameworks and evidence-informed strategies, it insists that antiracism must move beyond rhetoric into praxis, where theory meets deliberate, responsible, accountable sustained action.

The book is a challenge and a call to action. A challenge to practitioners, educators, leaders and policymakers to interrogate entrenched unjust norms, reimagine curricula and embed antiracism principles into healthcare systems' designs. It is an invitation to every reader to engage deeply, reflect honestly and act radically (meaning differently from the status quo). Antiracism is not a destination but a lifelong, reflexive journey, that demands humility and unwavering commitment to actionable change.

The book belongs on every shelf, whether you are a practitioner, an educator, a policymaker, leader or a member of the public who believes in justice-based healthcare. I have deep gratitude for the chapter authors and the editor whose vision and collaborations have made this work possible.

May the pages of the book inspire you not only to think differently but to be, do and lead differently. Let us together transform nursing and midwifery healthcare breaking away from its colonial chains into an authentically accountable, evidence-informed, inclusive, equitable and just system. The time for action is now.

Professor Sinegugu Duma
Dean of Teaching & Learning
College of Health Sciences
University of KwaZulu-Natal

PREFACE

You may want to know why an occupational therapist is editing a book on antiracism nursing and midwifery. Well .... My overall interest and writings are on antiracism approach and decolonising healthcare education. It felt natural and transferrable to work with peers in nursing and midwifery springboarding from my scholarly interest and expertise.

In the pages that follow, you will encounter a collective call to action, one that challenges the nursing and midwifery professions to confront their historical complicity in racism and to reimagine their futures through the perspective of antiracism. This book is not simply a compilation of chapters; it is an interconnection of critical scholarship, transformative praxis and sometimes lived experiences. This is brought to view by the chapter contributors from across the globe who are united in their commitment to justice, equity and liberation of nursing and midwifery. However, it does not pass me by the colonial pull, as our Brazilian contributors had to write in not their first language, but in English, to think, translate and compose in two languages is challenging. I am grateful they persevered.

As the editor, I am humbled to have the privilege of gathering voices that speak truth to power. These voices of nurses, midwives, educators, researchers and activists do not shy away from the uncomfortable. They interrogate the colonial legacies embedded in nursing and midwifery curricula, expose the systemic racism that persists in clinical practice and illuminate the structural barriers that Black and minoritised professionals and service users continue to face. They also instil hope through reimagining strategy and vision going forwards for antiracism change for a profession that can and must do better.

This book is grounded in the understanding that racism is here and now systemically within nursing and midwifery. From the erasure of Black and Indigenous pioneers to the marginalisation of internationally educated nurses, the profession has long upheld colonial systems that privilege whiteness. Yet, within this history lies the potential for radical transformation. By including antiracism approach, CRT, Critical Whiteness Studies and intersectional ideas, the chapters provide theoretical perspectives, analysis and evaluations and the practical pathways to move towards disruption to eventual dismantling of these oppressive structures.

This book is not for passive consumption; it is an invitation to co-create and co-produce actionable change. Hence each chapter concludes with a reflective activity based on Bain et al.'s 5R framework, with subheadings: Reporting, Responding, Relating, Reasoning and Reconstructing, for readers to engage deeply with the material and consider its implications for their own practice, pedagogy and leadership.

To those who have experienced racism within nursing and midwifery, you matter and your stories matter to keep chipping away at change. To the antiracism movers and shakers, to those already signed up for action, we are with you, keep going because you are on the right side of liberating this profession. To make sure we reduce the health disparities in nursing and midwifery by spotlighting and putting actions in place to remove them. For those just beginning, welcome and hurry up, this work is urgent.

Let this book be a mirror and guide for nursing and midwifery and motivate you to be a catalyst to move from rhetoric to reality for transformative health justice.

Dr Musharrat J. Ahmed-Landeryou, PhD
Editor
Associate Professor in Teaching and Learning
Professional Lead in Occupational Therapy
Deputy Head of the School of Allied Health and Life Sciences
London South Bank University

ACKNOWLEDGEMENTS

- My deepest gratitude goes to my husband and daughter, whose unwavering love have carried me through the long hours and emotional labour of education activism for antiracism and equity. For believing with me, as I do, that this work matters profoundly.
- High gratitude to the authors of the foreword and chapters for your generosity to join me and giving of your time shaped this book, without your words, insights and commitment, these pages simply would not exist.
- I am deeply appreciative of all those who I made meaningful and invaluable connections with along the way, introducing me to inspiring professionals, expanding my thinking and opening doors.
- Sincere thanks to the endorsers of this book, your willingness to review the book and to stand with us is essential in bringing this necessary and accessible work into the world.

Love and peace to all who walk this journey. Together, as a collective, we are stronger to challenge, disrupt and ultimately dismantle racism from healthcare.

1

WHAT IS RACISM DOING IN A NICE PROFESSION LIKE NURSING AND MIDWIFERY?

Natalie Stake-Doucet and Sarah Esegbona-Adeigbe

In this chapter concepts of racism and discrimination will be discussed and interpersonal, institutional and systemic racism explored. The historical origins of racism and discrimination in nursing and midwifery practice and an examination of how the ideological basis of racism was developed and embedded into the current worldview is provided. An overview of key Black and Indigenous figures in nursing and midwifery history and the discriminatory barriers and challenges that were experienced is undertaken, providing a picture of how racism and discrimination has filtered into current day practices. In addition, a brief inquiry into anti-racism in the current climate of nursing and midwifery practice is presented and the importance of creating a workplace that is just, equitable, and liberatory for nurses, midwives, other healthcare professionals, employees, and service users. This chapter will conclude with the lessons learnt from the history of racism and discrimination in contemporary nursing and midwifery practice.

Introduction

According to the World Health Organization (WHO) (2022): 'Racism is an ideological construct that assigns a certain race and/or ethnic group to a position of power over others on the basis of physical and cultural attributes, as well as economic wealth, involving hierarchical relations where the "superior" race exercises domination and control over others' (p.4). There are many definitions of the word 'racism', with different interpretations depending on the context in which it is used. The word racism is etymologically derived from the word 'race', which is a social, not a biological concept, that has no scientific basis. Race is the categorisation of groups of people based on shared physical and social characteristics; therefore, 'race' is a socially constructed human invention. An individual's race is determined

DOI: 10.4324/9781003565369-1

by perceived or learnt ideologies, which one could suggest is real (culture or ethnicity) or imaginary (intelligence or education). Racialised groups that are not White, and Indigenous groups are deemed to be inferior and are subjected to differential treatment in all walks of society, including healthcare. To be 'racist' is when one believes that one's own race makes one superior to others, rationalising the privileges of one's own race. Racism leads to disempowerment and the oppression and antagonism of individuals. It is also argued that racism continuously undergoes change, resulting in new forms of political, social, cultural, and linguistic expressions (Omi and Winant, 2014).

Racism can be individual, interpersonal, institutional, or systemic. Individual racism relates to a person's beliefs. It can be conscious or unconscious, whereas interpersonal racism relates to racist actions (microaggression), e.g., racist comments to the exclusion of opportunities. The extreme end of interpersonal racism can manifest as hate crimes towards individuals and/or communities. Institutional racism relates to the presence of racist policies, practices, and culture within an institution, such as a hospital or within a profession, for example, like in nursing and midwifery, which is the topic of this chapter. Finally, systemic/structural racism refers to the social organization of reward and privilege along racialised lines (Bonilla-Silva, 1997), e.g., laws, government organisation of funding. This chapter will address institutional and systemic racism as they relate to nursing and midwifery.

A Short History of Racism in Nursing

Caring for people is as old as humanity itself; and is arguably one of the defining traits of humanity. However, the care of fellow humans is not a static thing; it has evolved and changed as societies have progressed and regressed. Sociopolitical milestones and historical events have profoundly impacted care and health, from the discovery of antibiotics to colonization and the professionalization of various healthcare providers. The legacy of colonialism and the Transatlantic slave trade have had important consequences on the world that continue to be visible today. Nursing and midwifery, for example, despite being caring professions, are not exempt from perpetuating racism. Health sciences, like medicine and nursing, have a long history of racism towards Black and Indigenous people. For instance, the so-called father of gynaecology in the U.S. built his reputation and prestige through his experimentation and abuse of Black enslaved women (Nuriddin et al., 2020). Further racism was highlighted in America in the 1950s, when Henrietta Lacks was treated for cervical cancer in the only health facility that provided free healthcare for African Americans. During diagnosis and treatment, she had cells removed from her tumour without her consent, a common occurrence in segregated America. These cells were the first immortal cell line and have been used extensively for biomedical research. Her cells were used by scientists in the development of the first polio vaccine in the 1950s, and more recently, in the development of the COVID-19 mRNA vaccine. Her cells, taken without her knowledge or consent, or that of her family, have played an unprecedented role in medical research. Ms. Lacks died in 1951, but her cells live. Only recently has she begun to receive recognition for her contribution to science. It was only after more than 60 years of working to honour her legacy that her family finally obtained a central role in how and by whom her cells were used (John Hopkins University, 2024). The disregard for Lacks' privacy and dignity is evident, highlighting the discrimination that was present at the time (Clark, 2021).

In the U.K., another example of racism was the belief that migrants from Commonwealth countries had brought sickle cell into the U.K. Many people in the 1950s and 1960s held the belief that sickle cell was an infectious disease that Black nurses were passing onto White people, despite the scientific data that demonstrated it was an inherited, not infectious disease (Redhead,2022). These beliefs, steeped in xenophobic fearmongering, led to suggestions in parliament to prevent Black individuals from donating blood. Sickle cell patients were labelled as drug addicts, and dismissed and maltreated, an experience that is still evident today in the U.K. (Limb, 2025). These instances in history demonstrate how racism has been perpetuated through the years, impacting both nurses and service users.

Joyce Echaquan

In Canada in 2020, the death of Joyce Echaquan, a 37-year-old Attikamekw First Nation woman, drew international attention to the systemic barriers to health and care equity for First Nations, Inuit, and Métis people. Joyce Echaquan recorded the moments before her death with her cell phone, which revealed racist abuse by a nurse and an orderly. They ignored her calls for help and her respiratory distress. A subsequent inquest explicitly stated that systemic racism in healthcare was a contributing factor in her death (Kamel, 2021). While both the nurse and orderly in the video were eventually fired, her family and her Attikamekw community worked to develop a framework to address much more broadly the consequences of racism in healthcare. In 2020, the Council of the Atikamekw of Manawan introduced Joyce's Principle, a comprehensive statement and guide for all levels of government, professional colleges and teaching institutions to commit to respect the rights of Indigenous people in Quebec and Canada. It aims to 'establish relations free from systemic racism for Indigenous people and the health and social services systems in Quebec and Canada' (p. 6). While the principle had been adopted by many boards of healthcare and nursing organizations, the work of implementing in meaningful ways remains. The office of Joyce's Principle opened in 2020 to ensure accountability and follow-up from organizations that have adopted the principle, and to continue lobbying for its adoption at all levels of government (Council of the Attikamekw of Manawan, 2020).

Many health professions are slowly beginning to recognize the racist harm they have contributed to, and nursing is no exception. In 2020, for instance, the New

Zealand Nurses Organisation (NZNO) explained that they would no longer celebrate Florence Nightingale's birthday, designated as International Nurses' Day: 'It is now known that Nightingale supported the alienation of Mâori land, in order to force migration to European settlements … The continued veneration of Florence Nightingale … is disrespectful and painful. Raising her as the beacon for nursing globally causes trauma and re-ignites the history and pain of colonisation' (Brooks and Nuku, 2020, p. 34–35). The NZNO article underlined how nursing remains embedded in its racist history, and the harm it continues to wreak. In this section, we will provide an overview of racism in nursing, and its impact on patient care and on nurses themselves.

Systemic and Institutionalised Racism Within Nursing

In this section, we will explore systemic and institutional racism and how these phenomena are often embedded in the nursing profession. We will explore how the structure of professional organizations for nursing, like professional associations and colleges, contributed to the whitewashing of nursing history and the attempt to erase the presence of Black and Indigenous nurses.

Systemic Racism in Nursing

Systemic racism is the accumulation of 'long-term effects from inequities due to power and unequal opportunities across systems' (WHO, 2022, p. 4). In other words, systemic racism has far reaching impacts on every aspect of the lives of those who experience this. Systemic racism is built into social norms, mechanisms, and processes, and exists as self-actualising, regardless of the intentions of the individuals who work within these mechanisms and processes. It is a phenomenon with traceable economic, political, and social consequences. One of the easiest areas to cartograph systemic racism is within housing. Now, what does housing have to do with nursing? Aside from being an important social determinant of health, gatekeeping access to housing was also a way to exclude Black students from nursing schools (Manthey, 2020). Let us unpack an example from the United States:

In 1929, Frances Mchie, a young Black woman, applied to the University of Minnesota School of Nursing. Her initial application was rejected on the basis of her race, despite Minnesota having passed anti-discrimination legislation almost 50 years before. Part of the reason for her rejection was that there was no housing available for Black nursing students. Mchie fought for her admission into the school of nursing and eventually won. She was the first Black woman admitted to the University of Minnesota School of Nursing. However, because of segregated housing policies, she was forced to live far away from campus during the duration of her studies. She eventually graduated at the top of her class in 1932, but housing for Black students remained an important barrier to nursing studies well into the 1960s (Manthey, 2020).

The story of nurse pioneer Frances Mchie is echoed in the experience of Black nurses throughout the United States, Canada, and many countries in Europe. The interaction of federal and state governments, university administrations, and municipalities helped keep Black women from attending schools of nursing, while simultaneously shielding schools of nursing from accusations of racial discrimination. In Mchie's case, the school of nursing vehemently denied any discrimination, blaming instead hospital and university policies for their own refusal to admit her into the school. Cases like Mchie's abound in nursing history, with consequences for Black students that continue to be visible today.

To this day, racism continues to harm nurses and patients. In the U.S., for example, nearly two-thirds of Black nurses reported being passed over for promotions because of the color of their skin (Iheduru-Anderson et al., 2025). Nurses in Canada, the U.K., and elsewhere report similar experiences; for Black, Brown, Indigenous, and immigrant nurses, racism is often a daily reality (Baines, 2024; Baptiste et al., 2021; Brooks and Nuku, 2020). On a more global scale, the legacy of colonialism has entrenched White dominance in nursing education and practice, systematically marginalising voices from the Global South (Bell, 2021; Suárez-Baquero, 2024).

Institutional Racism in Nursing

Institutional racism is both a driver and a product of systemic racism. The WHO defines institutional racism as discriminatory attitudes and practices that are embedded in institutions (WHO, 2022). These can include educational, criminal justice, healthcare, political, and social welfare institutions, as well as private companies such as banks and corporations. Institutional racism stems from laws, regulations, policies, or power systems that disadvantage individuals based on their perceived race or ethnicity (WHO, 2022, p. 4).

Nursing is a professional institution, and in most countries around the world, there are professional colleges to deliver and monitor regulated nursing practice, or at the very least, formal laws and regulations that determine the content of nursing education, nursing activities, and scope of practice (WHO, 2022). Over decades, intensive lobbying efforts, organised by nursing, fought for the development of formal legislation to professionalize nursing work. This political process often included championing racist and discriminatory values and norms (Stake-Doucet, 2023). While many scholars of nursing have studied the devastating impacts of racism in nursing on patient outcomes, more and more research is looking at how institutional racism is built into professional nursing itself, a multifaceted phenomenon that impacts all nurses and patients through the intersections of oppressions on one hand, and unearned privilege on the other (Baptiste, 2015; Baptiste et al., 2021; Esegbona-Adeigbe, 2021; Iheduru-Anderson and Wahi, 2022). Institutional racism in nursing is a much more complex phenomenon than a few 'bad' nurses, and requires a broader understanding of nursing history and its relationship to slavery and colonial violence, and the political process of professionalization.

In her ground-breaking book, Black Women in White, Darlene Clark Hine details the genealogy of the various nursing groups and associations that led to the professionalization of nursing in the United States. While one may argue that the United States is different than in other countries, Hine's exhaustive historical research shows how nursing organizations aimed at professionalising nursing work were founded to include U.S. and Canadian White nurse leaders, who had sought the counsel of White British nurse leaders. The nursing leadership in all three countries collaborated in articulating a nursing ideal that was based on whiteness. Ethel Gordon Fenwick, the founder of the British Nurses' Association, for example, played a key role in establishing the Society of Superintendents of Training Schools for Nursing in the United States and Canada, which later evolved into the American Nurses Association (Hine, 2020). She goes on to explain how professionalization mostly benefitted White nurses, while increasing barriers to practice for Black nurses. Nursing organizations adhered to segregation laws, and in many states, professional organisations and nursing schools banned Black nurses from taking licensure exams, for example. In Canada, nursing schools refused admission to Black and Indigenous students until after World War II, much like in the U.K. (Flynn, 2011; McCallum, 2014).

The absence of Indigenous registered nurses in North America until the 20th century reflected genocide and the erasure of millennial health knowledge (Bourque-Bearskin, 2023). The caring and health work of Indigenous people was never recognised as such. The registration system of nursing favoured White nurses, who had studied in so-called 'modern' schools that rejected any health knowledge and traditions that were not rooted in 19th-century imperialist values and worldviews.

Human beings have always engaged in nursing care, but the standardization and professionalisation of nursing care in the 19th and 20th centuries in the U.S., U.K., and Canada only recognised as nurses those white women who fit their narrow definition of what a nurse should look like (DiGregorio, 2023, Flynn, 2014; Stake-Doucet, 2023).

Racism and Nursing Care

Racism in nursing is a result of both institutional and systemic racism. The following sections will offer a concrete perspective at institutional racism in nursing, by looking at the life and nursing work of Harriet Tubman, an American Civil War hero, and Edith Monture, the first Indigenous woman in Canada to be recognised as a registered nurse by nursing organisations there. Mary Seacole who played a pivotal role as a nurse who wanted to support the British during the Crimean war is also discussed and the nurses who responded to the call for healthcare workers during the Windrush era and after and the subsequent discrimination experienced in the U.K. Their lives and work are more than examples of institutional racism, they are role models for all nurses and their stories are a fundamental part of nursing history.

Harriet Tubman

Harriet Tubman is probably one of the most well-known heroes of the American civil war. While a few nursing organizations today honour her as part of nursing history, her years of working as a nurse for the Union army were not recognised until more than 30 years after the end of the war. For the first time, a woman was formally contracted by the U.S. Army; that woman was Dorothea Dix, appointed to be superintendent of army nurses. Dix was not a nurse, but a fervent admirer of Nightingale and a leading reformer (Gibbons-Backus, 2024). She refused to hire any Black or Catholic women into the army nursing corps, effectively banning some of the women who arguably had the most experience in nursing at the time. Her authority remained limited in the face of the bloody realities of war. Whether they were approved by Dix or not, many women simply showed up to be nurses, like Harriet Tubman (DiGregorio, 2023). Tubman's exploits are now common knowledge; she was a conductor on the Underground Railroad until 1861, when she joined the Union Army at the outbreak of the Civil War. Even at the time, her exploits made her famous and she was celebrated in the press. Despite her heroism and notoriety, nursing leaders like Dix would not recognize her as a nurse, despite Tubman doing all the work consistent with nursing.

Many of the people who had simply 'shown up' to nurse the Union Army in whatever capacity they could were left out of pension considerations after the war (DiGregorio, 2023). Furthermore, despite Dix's narrow view, the U.S. surgeon General at the time ended up going over Dix to recruit more nurses. The need for nurses was simply too vast to stick to Dix's bigoted criteria. In 1865, Tubman was appointed by the Surgeon General himself as nurse matron of Fort Monroe's Colored Hospital in Hampton. Harriet Tubman only received an army pension in 1899, after years of fighting for recognition of her service. Although her work and courage were undeniable, it took decades after her death before White dominated nursing associations looked beyond Dix to begin claiming Tubman as a nursing hero. While Tubman is widely celebrated as a civil war hero, her recognition as a nurse by nursing organizations remains inadequate. The inadequacy of her recognition within nursing is a problem for today that reflects ongoing tensions within nursing as to whom can be formally recognised as a nurse, especially when recognising a Black nurse could create conflict with the historically accepted legacy of professional nursing and the White women still being honoured for it.

Edith Monture

Edith Monture was the first Indigenous woman to be recognised as a registered nurse in Canada. Monture was born in 1890, on Haudenosaunee land, on the Six

Nations community in Ontario, Canada. When she finished high school, she applied to several nursing schools in Ontario, but never received a response (Eggertson, 2020). She was not deterred; she travelled to New York, where she attended the New Rochelle School of Nursing, graduating at the top of her class in 1914 (Conn, 2023). She was working as a school nurse in New Rochelle when the U.S. entered World War I in 1917. She volunteered and joined the U.S. Army Nursing Corps. She spent over a year based at military hospital in Vittel, France, but was often called to other hospitals and to walk the battlefields looking for injured soldiers. She detailed her experience in her war journal, which was published privately by her family in 1996. The diary gives us a glimpse of her experience as a wartime nurse. She writes of heartbreak when a patient who had 'adopted' her as his big sister died from a haemorrhage. She writes of busy days and idle days, of hearing bombs, of having to care for German prisoners. Very few nurse diaries of World War I have been preserved, and Monture's diary is the only one written by an Indigenous nurse. Despite her family having made her diary available online, Monture's writing is not required reading in nursing schools in Canada.

While Monture is often recognised today as the first Indigenous registered nurse in Canada, no nursing school or association recognizes how nursing itself made it so difficult for her to become a registered nurse in the first place. Furthermore, it essentializes Indigenous nursing to the parts that are recognised by a colonial and racist system. Historian Mary-Jane Logan McCallum explains that looking at the 'first' Indigenous nurse 'relies on modern institutional and professional definitions of "nurse" that are exclusive of the range of health work in which Indigenous people have historically engaged' (p. 254). While learning about Edith Monture should be the norm in nursing school, the work to recognize and acknowledge professional nursing's role in the ongoing genocide against Indigenous people in North America remains undone.

Mary Seacole

One of the Black icons of British nursing was Mary Seacole, a Jamaican-born nurse who travelled to England in 1854 to seek permission to care for British soldiers during the Crimean War but was turned down. Seacole overcame racism and injustices during this time and funded her own travels to Crimea and set up a British hotel to care for sick soldiers (Royal College of Nurses, 2024). Seacole was well known as Florence Nightingale at the time, and soldiers wrote letters of support praising her work. Seacole was actually in Crimea, on the front lines, whereas Nightingale worked from Constantinople, some 300 miles away (Nagai, 2004). However, she was lost to history for over a century. In 2004, Seacole was voted the greatest Black Briton (Ono-George, 2022). This recognition was long overdue, highlighting the double standard between her and Nightingale work. Whilst Nightingale was given uninterrupted accolades for 100 years, the same recognition was not given to Seacole. Eventually, after more than a decade of campaigning by the Mary Seacole Trust, a statue in her honour was erected in the grounds of St Thomas Hospital in London in 2016 (Mary Seacole Trust, 2023). Seacole's work has now justly received recognition and accolades but discussions about how racism had impacted her legacy, and how to dismantle the institutional and systemic racism that was faced by those working to honour her legacy is much less discussed.

The Windrush Nurses

Further examples of racism in U.K. nursing are evident from the Windrush era. Mass immigration from the Commonwealth was a solution to a shortage of nurses and midwives in the U.K. National Health Service in the 1940s. British citizenship was granted to individuals from British colonies and former British colonies. A change in the National Health Service (NHS) workforce was evident with more diverse nurses providing care. Prejudice, stereotyping, and discrimination became evident with the increased presence of nurses from Africa, the Caribbean, and other Commonwealth countries. Mass immigration from the Commonwealth was criticised in 1968 due to xenophobic fears and presumed lack of integration of immigrants. Nurses from the Commonwealth countries were treated poorly and not offered equal opportunities for promotion. Daphne Steele, was the first Black matron in the NHS, known to push boundaries and advocate for change in a system that treated Black and minority ethnic nurses unequally. Steele experienced challenges but despite this worked hard and remained dedicated leading to promotion. The NHS faced further shortages in nursing, with the popularity of the profession declining in the 1980s, partly due to the abolition of work permits for overseas nurses. Due to the expansion of the NHS in 2000, leading to additional demand, recruitment of workers from India began (Snow and Jones, 2011). However, recruited overseas trained nurses had to undergo a programme of supervised practice, with many facing discrimination and exploitation, and their skills and experiences not being recognised. Racism has continued to infiltrate U.K. nursing, acknowledged by the RCN (2024), stating that 32% of nurses and 10.7% of health visitors are Black, but they continue to face challenges and abuse in a system that prevents equal opportunity. Despite the RCN championing equity, diversity, and inclusion, racism is alive and well in the U.K. nursing profession.

Racism in the Midwifery Profession

As long as women have been giving birth they have been supported by other women (Staras, 2022). Glimpses into the history of midwifery show the presence of Black and Indigenous midwives. The following section discusses racism in midwifery across different contexts and how this has impacted on the profession and the childbearing population.

Racism in American Midwifery

During colonial times in the U.S.A., midwives supported women in childbirth amongst the Indigenous people and the traditional midwifery practices from Africa were present due to the Transatlantic slave trade. Enslaved African women were known as granny midwives and cared for enslaved women during childbirth, but also attended to White women. After emancipation, granny midwives continued to work with both White and Black women, as hospitals were rarely accessible in the mid-19th century. However, with the development of the field of obstetrics, Black midwifery was attacked and replaced. White medical practitioners wanted to protect their status in the field of childbirth and so deemed granny and other Indigenous midwives as being unsafe and causing maternal mortality. In the early 1800s, many American states created laws that prohibited granny midwives. There are reports of African American midwives being gradually racially ousted of practice in the late-20th century through health care initiatives (Craven and Glatzel, 2010). The term nurse-midwife was coined in 1914, to differentiate between nurses educated in midwifery and immigrant and African American midwives who did not have the same sort of training.

At the 20th Annual Convention of the American Nurses' Association in 1917, a gynaecologist was invited to give a keynote address on what nursing leaders called 'the midwife problem'. In his speech, he stated: 'The midwife is an undesirable product of foreign immigration' (Davis, 1917, p. 970). This type of discourse within nursing and medicine set the tone for an organised campaign against traditional midwifery that lasted for decades. Between 1900 and 1940, health officials and medical doctors depicted granny and immigrant midwives as an illegitimate health care providers (Bonaparte, 2023). Hence, begun the dark era of systematic eradication of African-American and immigrant midwives. By the 1940s, Black women were required to undertake training and be licensed to undertake midwifery. Licenses were under the purview of white nurses and physicians, which resulted in the elimination of granny midwives and the creation of nurse midwives (Niles and Drew, 2020; Shead, 2022). Black midwives were systematically excluded from midwifery practice, a historical wrong that has impacted the midwifery profession until the present day.

The presence of Black midwives was crucial for Black and immigrant women, as often they could not afford the cost of hospital care or White doctors, and were rightfully apprehensive of the racist treatment they would likely receive.

Margaret Charles Smith was the first Black traditional midwife in the U.S. with a permit in the state of Alabama. She delivered over 3000 babies between 1949 to 1976 (Weig-Pickering, 2022). Smith experienced racism during her years of midwifery practice, however mothers and babies lives were saved. This is significant as at the time Black midwives were depicted as being illiterate, lazy, and incompetent. Black midwives were subjected to scorn whilst their White counterparts received respect.

One of the most well-known figures in midwifery in the U.S.A. is Mary Breckinridge. Nursing and midwifery literature recognize her as a nurse leader who opened the first midwifery school in the U.S.A. in 1939 (Ulrich et al., 2013). What is less known about her is that she was politically active White supremacist. The school she founded is now known as the Frontier Nursing University. In 2019, at the request of concerned students, a taskforce was established to look into Breckinridge's racist history (Mary Breckinridge Task Force, 2020). Very quickly, it became clear the students had every reason to be concerned. For nearly 30 years the school refused to admit Black students; not until Breckenridge's death in 1965 (Canadian Association of Midwives, 2021; Niles and Drew, 2020). There were no midwifery schools when this school was founded; most midwives were Black, Indigenous, or immigrant women who had learned through traditional training that often carried millennia of knowledge. Breckinridge's school did not recognize the traditional or 'granny' midwives and Breckinridge contributed to their demonization. The school admitted only nurse graduates, in a conscious attempt to whitewash midwifery and undermine traditional midwifery. Breckinridge was an influential player in the eradication of midwifery traditions that had been transmitted for centuries, millennia even, yet she remains revered today as a 'savior' of midwifery and pioneer of women's health (Michel, 2024; Niles and Drew, 2020; Tate, 2016). In the U.S.A. today, the midwifery profession is dominated by White midwives and does not reflect the ethnic identities of the population served (Mehra et al., 2023). Black, Hispanic, American Indian, or Alaska Natives account for less than 20% of the midwifery profession (Mehra et al., 2022). Potential barriers to the midwife profession are interpersonal and institutionalised racism, leading to feelings of otherness and not belonging to the profession (Kennedy et al., 2006; Craft-Blacksheare and Kahn, 2023).

Indigenous women in Canada are disproportionately subjected to maltreatment due to systemic racism, which is attributed to the impact of colonialism (Tomkins et al., 2024).

Racism in Canadian Midwifery

Erosion oflIndigenous midwives and control of their knowledge and practices was the result of colonization in Canada. The history of midwifery in Canada does not acknowledge Indigenous midwives; instead, European midwives are recorded from the 17th century, erasing the centuries of knowledge held by Indigenous birth attendants (Relyea, 1992). Subsequently, Western birthing practices were widespread across Canada, whilst Indigenous birthing practices were deemed inferior and uncivilised (Murdock and Durant, 2024). Indigenous peoples faced racist and discriminatory practices from settler midwives, who were unable to provide culturally appropriate care or meet their individual needs. Midwifery regulation begun in the 1990s in Canada (National Aboriginal Council of Midwives, 2016) and racism arising from Canadian health law and health policies on Indigenous communities increased erosion of Indigenous identities (Cohen-Fournier et al., 2021). Midwifery education programmes maintained colonialism by utilising Western practices to suppress the growth of Indigenous midwifery. In 2020, an independent review commissioned by the Minister of Health found evidence of systemic racism in the British Columbia healthcare system (Aerts et al., 2024). Systematic and interpersonal racism reported in Ontario midwifery (Aseffa et al., 2024), has contributed to the oppression of Indigenous midwives. It is also stated that reproductive healthcare is used as a tool to control and subjugate Indigenous people and to advance the White settler state (Murdock and Durant, 2024). The Canadian Association of Midwives (2021) recognised that Indigenous midwifery was a protected force against racism in health care settings, leading to investments into eliminating anti-Indigenous racism in Canada.

Racism in U.K. Midwifery

Midwives have been present in the U.K. since the 1500s and were legally recognised in Britain in 1902 with the first Midwives Act. Similar to nursing, Black and minority ethnic midwives began to enter the U.K. during the Windrush era, encouraged due to the post-World War I baby boom. However, Black women faced barriers to undertaking midwifery training, often relegated to State Enrolled Nurses (SEN) a qualification with less recognition than the State Registered Nurse (SRN). Nursing authorities at the time believed that their race limited their intellectual abilities to undergo SRN training (Snow and Jones, 2011). This limited their career progression to undertake midwifery training, as a requirement was to be an SRN. Recruitment of young women from abroad continued in the U.K., with an estimated 10,566 students having been recruited by 1972 (Snow and Jones, 2011). However, non-White midwives are poorly represented in senior positions in the NHS and are more likely to be referred to the regulatory body, the Nursing and Midwifery Council (NMC) (RCN, 2021). In the present day, the Royal College of Midwives (RCM) state that midwives of non-White ethnicity are more likely to experience bullying, harassment, and discrimination in the workplace and are likely to face disciplinary proceedings (RCN, 2021).

Furthermore, non-White midwives were less likely to have career progression and opportunities for promotion. Racism has crept into midwifery practice, recognised by Birthrights as being at the root of inequities in maternity care (Birthrights, 2022). Black and brown women are almost four times more likely to die during pregnancy and childbirth and have a stillbirth compared to White women in most countries worldwide (Felker et al., 2024). Black and Brown women have been at increased risk of dying during pregnancy since 2000, showing the depth and breadth of the issue. Discriminatory practices and microaggressions in maternity services are alluded to in U.K. maternal mortality reports, and case reviews into maternal deaths frequently state that a different outcome may have occurred if appropriate care had been provided (Felker et al., 2024). A profession that started out to provide a supporting and comforting environment during childbirth has now become a place of fear and dread for some women. Furthermore, Black and Brian midwives in the U.K. have to tackle racist and discriminatory practices on a regular basis.

A Brief Enquiry into Anti-Racist Practices

The importance of anti-racist practices has been highlighted by a brief look into the nursing and midwifery experiences of Black, Brown, and Indigenous nurses and midwives. Overwhelmingly, the obvious barriers created by systemic and institutional racism and discrimination demonstrate the impact on the quality of healthcare provision and the negative consequences for healthcare professionals and service users. Many healthcare organisations globally have produced anti-racist policies and mandates, which are often seen as insignificant and performative (RCN, 2021; Montague et al., 2025). The invisibility of Black, Brown, and Indigenous knowledge birthed by colonialism and reared by racism and discrimination has fed institutional and systemic racism in the nursing and midwifery professions. There has been denial about racist practices in nursing and midwifery professions and limited attention to these issues in nursing and midwifery training programmes (Playfair et al., 2023). Moreover, despite the COVID-19 pandemic highlighting institutional racism globally, recognition of the colonial impact on Black, Brown, and Indigenous nurses and midwives' experiences remains limited (Prendergast, 2024). To ignore the impact of colonialism on the nursing and midwifery professions and the role Black, Brown, and Indigenous nurses and midwives have played in this arena highlights the real problems at hand. Such silencing does not aid the eradication of racism, nor does it assists in anti-racist policies and strategies. Hence, racist and discriminatory practices are likely to continue, unheeded and unfettered. Herein lies the undeniable truth that until there is a robust acceptance of racism in the nursing and midwifery professions and its impact on Black, Brown, and Indigenous healthcare professionals, the next 50 to 100 years will portray a similar picture.

Lessons Learned from History for Anti-Racist Nursing and Midwifery Today

So how do we learn from the history of nursing and midwifery to ensure the future is on a different, more just and accountable path? With this chapter, we take the first step. Recognising how nursing and midwifery, as they exist today in countries of the Global North, reflect the violence of racism and colonialism on which they were primarily built. The first step towards anti-racist nursing and midwifery professions must be to understand the truth of our professional history, and to understand and acknowledge the historical wrongs. Throughout this book, you will read about different contexts and ways of anti-racism actions in nursing and midwifery that will inspire your own practice to operationalise an anti-racism approach to nursing and midwifery. At the end of each of the chapters we ask you to pause and reflect using Bain et al.'s (2002) framework on what does what you read mean for your context and how to change. We must know and understand history to avoid its repetition, but beyond history, this book aims to provide inspiration and tools for nurses and midwives to dismantle the racism that exists within these professions.

Reflective Activity

Having read the chapter, we invite you to reflect on your key learning and its implications for your professional practice as a nurse or midwife using Bain et al.'s (2002) 5R framework (p. 13–15):

- Reporting – What is it in your situation you want to transform after reading this chapter?
- Responding – What are your personal observations regarding your own situation/context in relation to what is raised in this chapter?
- Relating – What is/are the theoretical/research/data/legislative, etc., understandings relationship to under consideration in this chapter that you could apply to your situation/context?
- Reasoning – Identify how the chapter findings matter to your situation/context and how will you interrogate your situation/context and what will help you from this chapter?
- Reconstructing – Identify your action plans to reframe and rebuild a transformative way forward to change from the situation in your context.

References

Aerts, L., Kwunuhmen, J.G., Johansen, C. and Luke, S. (2024). A continuous journey: Addressing IndigenousIndigenous-specific racism as a nursing and midwifery regulator. *Journal of Nursing Regulation, 15*(3): 47–53. https://www.journalofnursingregulation.com/article/S2155-8256(24)00074-7/fulltext

Aseffa, F., Mehari, L., Gure, F. and Ahmed, S. (2024). Disrupting racism in Ontario midwifery. *Journal of Midwifery & Women's Health, 69*(1): 52–57. https://doi.org/10.1111/jmwh.13541

Bain, J.D., Ballantyne, R., Mills, C. and Lester, N.C. (2002). *Reflecting on practice: Students teachers' perspectives*. Post Pressed.

Baines, E. (2024). Racism remains part of NHS culture, researchers warn. *Nursing Times*. https://www.nursingtimes.net/workforce/racism-remains-part-of-nhs-culture-researchers-warn-20-02-2024/

Baptiste, D.L., Turner, S., Josiah, N., Arscott, J., Alvarez, C., Turkson-Ocran, R.A., Rodney, T., Commodore-Mensah, Y., Francis, L., Wilson, P.R. and Starks, S. (2021). Hidden figures of nursing: The historical contributions of Black nurses and a narrative for those who are unnamed, undocumented and underrepresented. *Journal of Advanced Nursing, 77*(4): 1627–1632. https://doi.org/10.1111/jan.14791

Baptiste, M. (2015). Workplace discrimination: An additional stressor for internationally educated nurses. *The Online Journal of Issues in Nursing (OJIN), 20*(3): 8. https://doi.org/10.3912/OJIN.Vol20No03PPT01

Bell, B. (2021). White dominance in nursing education: A target for anti-racist efforts. *Nursing Inquiry*, *28*(1): e12379. https://doi.org/10.1111/nin.12379

Birthrights. (2022). *Systemic racism, not broken bodies: An inquiry into racial justice and human rights in UK maternity care*. Birthrights

Bonaparte, A.D. (2023). Regulating Childbirth: Physicians and Granny Midwives in South Carolina. In Alicia D. Bonaparte and Julia Chinyere Oparah (Eds.), *Birthing justice: Black women, pregnancy, and childbirth* (pp. 30–42). Routledge.

Bonilla-Silva, E. (1997). Rethinking racism: Toward a structural interpretation. *American Sociological Review*, *62*(3): 465–480. https://www.jstor.org/stable/2657316

Bonilla-Silva, E. (2021). What makes systemic racism *systemic*? *Sociological Inquiry*, *91*(3): 513–533. https://doi.org/10.1111/soin.12420

Brooks, G. and Nuku, K. (2020). Why we aren't celebrating Florence's birthday. *Kai Tiaki Nursing New Zealand*, *26*(3): 34–35.

Canadian Association of Midwives. (2021). *Combatting Anti-Indigenous Racism*. https://canadianmidwives.org/sites/canadianmidwives.org/wp-content/uploads/2022/03/CAM_PSCombattingAnti-IndigenousRacism_VF_20211020-1.pdf

Clark, M.J. (2021). Have hope: HeLa cells reveal the possibility and brokenness of our world. *US Catholic*, *86*(4): 40–42. https://www.thefreelibrary.com/Have%20hope:%20HeLa%20cells%20reveal%20the%20possibility%20and%20brokenness%20of%20our…-a0668968401

Cohen-Fournier, S.M., Brass, G. and Kirmayer, L.J. (2021). Decolonizing health care: Challenges of cultural and epistemic pluralism in medical decision-making with Indigenous-Indigenous communities. *Bioethics*, *35*(8): 767–778. https://doi.org/10.1111/bioe.12946

Conn, H. (2023). Edith Monture. *L'Encyclopédie Canadienne*. https://www.thecanadianencyclopedia.ca/fr/article/edith-monture

Council of the Atikamekw of Manawan. (2020). *Joyce's Principle*. https://principedejoyce.com/sn_uploads/principe/Joyce_s_Principle_brief___Eng.pdf

Craft-Blacksheare, M. and Kahn, P. (2023). Midwives' and other perinatal health workers' perceptions of the Black maternal mortality crisis in the United States. *Journal of Midwifery & Women's Health*, *68*(1): 62–70. https://doi.org/10.1111/jmwh.13433

Craven, C. and Glatzel, M. (2010). Downplaying difference: Historical accounts of African American midwives and contemporary struggles for midwifery. *Feminist Studies*, *36*(2): 330–358. http://www.jstor.org/stable/27919104

DiGregorio, S. (2023). *Taking Care: The Story of Nursing and Its Power to Change Our World*. HarperCollins.

Eggertson, L. (2020). Discrimination in Canada led First Nations nurse to train in New York to serve with U.S. https://community.cna-aiic.ca/blogs/cn-content/2020/11/09/discrimination-in-canada-led-first-nations-nurse-t

Esegbona-Adeigbe, S. (2021). The impact of a eurocentric curriculum on racial disparities in maternal health. *European Journal of Midwifery*, *5*(36). https://doi.org/10.18332/ejm/140086

Flynn, K.C. (2011). *Moving Beyond Borders: A History of Black Canadian and Caribbean Women in the Diaspora*. University of Toronto Press.

Gibbons-Backus, P. (2024). Dorothea Dix: Reformer, Author, Teacher, Nurse. *American Battlefield Trust*. https://www.battlefields.org/learn/articles/dorothea-dix-reformer-author-teacher-nurse

Hine, D.C., McCluskey, J. and Gaspar, D.B. (Eds.) (2020). *Black Women in White*. Indiana University Press.

Iheduru-Anderson, K., Waite, R. and Murray, T.A. (2025). The bastardization of DEIA: Regressing decades of progress in nursing and healthcare. *Nursing Inquiry*, *3*: e70027. https://doi.org/10.1111/nin.70027

Iheduru-Anderson, K.C. and Wahi, M.M. (2022). Race and racism discourse in U.S. nursing: Challenging the silence. *OJIN: The Online Journal of Issues in Nursing*, *27*(1) (Manuscript 1). https://www.doi.org/10.3912/OJIN.Vol27No01Man01

Johns Hopkins University. (2024). Johns Hopkins breaks ground on building named in honor of Henrietta Lacks. *The Hub*. https://hub.jhu.edu/2024/10/28/henrietta-lacks-building-groundbreaking-ceremony/

Kamel, G. (2021). Rapport d'enquête concernant le décès de Joyce Echaquan 2020-00275: Loi sur la recherche des causes et des circonstances des décès. *Québec: Bureau du Coroner*. https://www.coroner.gouv.qc.ca/fileadmin/contenu/Enqu%C3%AAtes_publiques/Joyce_Echaquan/2020-EP00275-9.pdf

Kennedy, H.P., Erickson-Owens, D. and Davis, J.A.P. (2006). Voices of diversity in midwifery: A qualitative research study. *Journal of Midwifery & Women's Health, 51*(2): 85–90. https://doi.org/10.1016/j.jmwh.2005.07.007

Limb, M. (2025). Sickle cell: Patients face 'systemic inequities' in care and research investments. *BMJ, 389*: r1274. https://doi.org/10.1136/bmj.r1274

Manthey, M. (2020). A history of systemic racism at the University of Minnesota School of Nursing. *Creative Nursing, 26*(3): 215–218. https://doi.org/10.1891/CRNR-D-20-00039

Mary Seacole Trust. (2023). *Memorials—Life, Work & Achievements of Mary Seacole*. https://www.maryseacoletrust.org.uk/memorials/

McCallum, M.J.L. (2014). *Indigenous women, work, and history: 1940–1980*. University of Manitoba Press.

Mehra R., Alspaugh A., Joseph J., Golden, B., Lanshaw, N., Mclemore, M.R., Frank, L.S. (2023). Racism is a motivator and a barrier for people of color aspiring to become midwives in the United States. *Health Services Research*, 58(1): 40–50 https://doi.org/10.1111/1475-6773.14037

Michel, A. (2024). The history of midwifery in the United States. *The Journal of Perinatal & Neonatal Nursing, 38*(2): 122–123. https://doi.org/10.1097/jpn.0000000000000812

Montague, J., Caxaj, C.S. and Webster, F. (2025). Call to action: Integrating anti-racist philosophies in dismantling racism and anti-black racism in nursing education in Canada. *Canadian Journal of Nursing Research, 57*(1): 112–126. https://doi.org/10.1177/08445621241296654

Murdock, M. and Durant, S. (2024). Settler midwifery: A colonial tool in Canada's reproductive healthcare system. *Birth (Berkeley, Calif.), 52*(3): 370–375. https://doi.org/10.1111/birt.12888

Niles, P.M. and Drew, M. (2020). *Constructing the modern American midwife: White supremacy and White feminism collide. Nursing Clio, Beyond Florence*. https://nursingclio.org/2020/10/22/constructing-the-modern-american-midwife-white-supremacy-and-white-feminism-collide/

Nuriddin, A., Mooney, G. and White, A.I.R. (2020). Reckoning with histories of medical racism and violence in the USA. *The Lancet, 396*(10256): 949–51. https://www.thelancet.com/action/showPdf?pii=S0140-6736%2820%2932032-8

Omi, M. and Winant, H. (2014). *Racial formation in the United States*. Routledge.

Playfair, C., Hunt, G. and DaCosta, C. (2023). Developing anti-racist undergraduate nursing education: Themes and action. *British Journal of Nursing, 32*(15): 736–742. https://www.britishjournalofnursing.com/content/professional/developing-anti-racist-undergraduate-nursing-education-themes-and-action

Prendergast, N. (2024). Ain't I a Nurse', implementing a digital illustration of resistance when challenging anti-Black racism in nursing education. *Nursing Philosophy, 25*(4): e12494. https://doi.org/10.1111/nup.12494

Redhead, G. (2022). *Empire, racism and the NHS: The history of sickle cell disorder*. Royal College of Nursing Magazine.

Relyea, M.J. (1992). The rebirth of midwifery in Canada: An historical perspective. *Midwifery, 8*(4): 159–169. https://doi.org/10.1016/s0266-6138(05)80002-6

Royal College of Nurses. (2024). *Nursing in the UK: Celebrating our diverse past, present and future*. https://www.rcn.org.uk/magazines/Opinion/2024/Oct/Nursing-in-the-UK-celebrating-our-diverse-past-present-and-future

Shead, S. (2022). Granny midwife to nurse-midwife: The decline of Southern Black midwifery in the 20th century. *Historical Perspectives: Santa Clara University Undergraduate Journal of History, Series II, 27*(1): 9. https://scholarcommons.scu.edu/historical-perspectives/vol27/iss1/9

Snow, S.J. and Jones, E.L. (2011). Immigration and the National Health Service: Putting history to the forefront. *History and Policy*. https://historyandpolicy.org/policy-papers/papers/immigration-and-the-national-health-service-putting-history-to-the-forefron/

Stake-Doucet, N. (2023). White privilege and professionalization: A decolonial and critical feminist perspective on professional nursing. *Witness: The Canadian Journal of Critical Nursing Discourse, 5*(2): 26–38. https://doi.org/10.25071/2291-5796.153

Staras, T. (2022). A brief history of district midwifery. *AIMS Journal: Once Upon a Birth, 34*(3): 12. https://issuu.com/aims1/docs/journal_34-3_final

Suárez-Baquero, D.F.M. (2024). Decolonizing nursing knowledge: Challenging eurocentrism centering global South voices. *Nursing Outlook, 72*(4): 102197. https://doi.org/10.1016/j.outlook.2024.102197

Tate, D.M. (2016). Mary Breckinridge: Angel on Horseback. In D.A. Forrester (Ed.), *Nursing's greatest leaders* (pp. 223–244). Springer Publishing Company. https://doi.org/10.1891/9780826130082.0010

Tomkins, S., Liu, J. and Campbell, L.A. (2024). Meaningful positioning: Insights on the importance of culturally safe, anti-racist settler-IndigenousIndigenous relationships in supporting IndigenousIndigenous maternal health in Canada. *International Journal of Indigenous Health, 19*(1) https://doi.org/10.32799/IJIH.V19I1.41140

Ulrich, S., Arthur, R. and Marfell, J. (2013). Outcomes Measurement in Nurse Midwifery Practice. In R.M. Kleinpell (Ed.), *Outcome assessment in advanced practice nursing* (pp. 203–219). Springer.

Weig-Pickering, A. (2022). 20220216_Margaret Charles Smith—An Extraordinary Midwife. https://libguides.health.unm.edu/blogs/hslic/Margaret-Charles-Smith-An-Extraordinary-Midwife-92117

World Health Organisation (WHO). (2020). *State of the world's nursing 2020: Investing in education, jobs and leadership*. World Health Organization. https://www.who.int/publications/i/item/9789240003279

World Health Organisation (WHO). (2022). *Strengthening primary health care to tackle racial discrimination, promote intercultural services and reduce health inequities: Research brief*. World Health Organization. https://www.who.int/publications/i/item/9789240057104

2

CRITICAL THEORIES TO DISRUPT RACISM IN NURSING AND MIDWIFERY

Critical Race Theory, Critical Whiteness Studies

Ifrah Salih and Musharrat J. Ahmed-Landeryou

Introduction

Racism within institutional systems persists despite decades of diversity initiatives and equal opportunity policies. Traditional approaches to addressing racialised inequality often focus on surface-level interventions that fail to examine the deeper structural foundations that perpetuate discriminatory outcomes. To move beyond these limitations, a more rigorous analytical framework is required—one that can penetrate the complex layers of systemic oppression and illuminate the mechanisms through which racial hierarchies are maintained and reproduced. This chapter will answer the *critical question:* how can Critical Race Theory (CRT) and Critical Whiteness Studies (CWS) help to disrupt racism in the nursing profession and education?

CRT and CWS offer powerful theoretical lenses for understanding how racism operates within institutional contexts. These frameworks move beyond individual prejudice to examine the ways in which policies, practices and organisational cultures systematically advantage some racial groups while disadvantaging others. Rather than treating racism as a result of individual bias, CRT and CWS position it as a fundamental organising principle embedded within the structure of institutions themselves.

The application of these theoretical constructs through systematic case study analysis provides a methodology for uncovering the often invisible mechanisms of racial oppression. By examining specific instances of discrimination, exclusion and differential treatment through the analytical frameworks of CRT and CWS, we can begin to map systemic racism and identify the points of intervention necessary for meaningful change. This approach moves away from anecdotal evidence or isolated incidents to develop a comprehensive understanding of how racism functions as a system of power relations.

DOI: 10.4324/9781003565369-2

Through the systematic application of CRT and CWS to real-world nursing case studies, we can develop more sophisticated understandings of how racism operates and, consequently, more effective strategies for dismantling it.

Expectations of Nurses and Midwives

Nurses and midwives abide by and follow the Nursing and Midwifery Code of Conduct (Nursing and Midwifery Council (NMC), 2018), which encompasses many expectations and behaviours demonstrated by nurses and midwives. One of the expectations is that nurses and midwives treat everyone equally, regardless of age, sex, race, etc. Nurses and midwives possess strong beliefs that they are non-racist as they are part of the nursing profession and view themselves as fair and non-judgmental (Symenuk et al., 2020). Discussing racialised inequalities in healthcare or within nursing represents a significant challenge, as no nurse believes they are racist or discriminatory (Bennett et al., 2019).

Reviewing Racism in Nursing and Midwifery through Critical Race Theory

CRT emerged from the mid-1970s in the USA among lawyers, activists and legal scholars due to the pace of racial reform and the effects of race and subtle forms of racism within the USA. This led to a movement within law (Delgado, 1995; Delgado & Stefancic, 2017). CRT analyses the effect of race within groups, which are deemed to be marginalised, resulting in social disparities (Ladson-Billings & Tate, 1995). Matsuda et al. (1993) further describe CRT as working towards "Eliminating racial oppression as part of the broader goal of ending all forms of oppression" (Matsuda et al., 1993, p. 6). Racial oppression is complex and often viewed as sensitive in nature in comparison to tackling other forms of oppression. Therefore, eliminating racism will support the eradication of other oppressive structures that exist.

Hiraldo (2010) describes CRT as critical studies that analyses and address racialised inequalities and is normally formed by a group of individuals who want to challenge and improve the relationship between racialised communities and power in different areas. Since the development of CRT, the concept has spread within education to explore biological racism within American schools and now it has become a global issue explored further afield including in the UK. In the UK, Higher Education Institutions (HEIs) are more than ever working towards being more diverse and inclusive and CRT can play a vital role in supporting this agenda. However, this approach is normally broad in nature and therefore fails to tackle the specificity of racism. Decuir and Dixson (2004) suggest that CRT was first used as an analytical framework back in 1994. Since then, CRT has been used to critique educational practice (Ladson-Billings, 2005) and is used to identify and analyse cultural and structural facets (Solórzano & Yosso, 2002). This includes teaching and learning practices, research to analyse practices using CRT and storytelling as well as campus environments. A further example of this across the sector is how higher education admission policies disadvantage Black applicants. This has led to higher education institutes creating widening participation initiatives to improve statistics, which led to them failing to address the structural barriers that exist as the disparities continue.

CRT is based on the premise that racism is embedded structurally and institutionally and then it impacts on the success of Minoritised people (Demathews & Watson, 2020).

CRT is made up of five tenets: counter-storytelling; permanence of racism; whiteness as a property; interest convergence; and the critique of liberalism (McCoy, 2006; Solórzano, 1997).

First tenant, counter-storytelling is simply explained as the narrative of the experiences of the Minoritised population. It's creating spaces for Minoritised people to have a voice to share their experiences of racism by recentering their voices and not of those who possess power, to resist and disrupt the status quo. Storytelling allows for dialogue, which perpetuates racism to be critiqued (Decuir & Dixson, 2004) and to challenge the beliefs that exist (Solórzano & Yosso, 2001). The voices need to be heard to set a story opposing the accepted righteousness of whiteness.

The second tenant permanence of racism is the suggestion that racism controls politics, social and economic aspects of society. This means that White individuals are privileged over Minoritised individuals systemically. Often preferential access, treatment or structures are invisible and unintentional (Gillborn, 2015). These structures advantaged White people to have power and control within various settings, known as White supremacy (Gillborn, 2015). White supremacy is the belief that White people are the superior race over all other races.

The third tenet, whiteness as a property, is the right to property, albeit whether it is the right of possession, enjoyment, disposition, or exclusion (Ladson-Billings, 1998). Harris (1993) adds an additional layer by explaining that this also incorporates ethnically minoritised people's self-identity and the structural advantages that they do not possess. Whiteness as a property is the right to a White identity and all the values that come with being White.

The fourth tenet is interest convergence, which was conceptualised by Bell Jr (1980) and proposes that change only occurs if the primary beneficiaries of legislation, policies and guidelines are White individuals rather than people who are Minoritised. Policies within organisations require a review using a CRT, anti-racist lens to explore who the main beneficiaries of such policies are. For example, policies reporting racial incidents on placements need to be open, transparent and created using CRT. This is to ensure that Minoritised students are able to report incidents and receive appropriate support, from this action demonstrating it benefits all. As the pull of whiteness dominates in the systems and policies tending to deny or diminish the racism issue/harm and CRT is a counteraction to disrupt the status quo.

The final and fifth tenet is the critique of liberalism and easily explained by the term colour blindness. A concept where White individuals claim that they do not see colour, and everyone is treated the same. However, claiming that you cannot see the skin colour of individuals perpetuates racism and the message received is that individuals do not recognise the daily barriers, exclusions and structural advantages that exist for EM students (McGibbon et al., 2014; Thorne, 2017).

The thrust of CRT is to challenge racism and to support the exploration of racialised bias by using a racialised equity lens and highlighting how racism impacts social structures and discourse (Browne et al., 2018).

Critical Race Theory in Nursing and Midwifery

The application of CRT to nursing remains understudied, as the field has only recently begun to acknowledge and examine the barriers faced by Minoritised nurses and midwives. Research exploring these challenges is still in its early stages and progressing gradually. CRT acknowledges that the experiences of Minoritised communities are important in understanding racialised discrimination, inequities and injustices that they face, rather than attempting to silence those experiences (Solorzano & Solorzano, 1995). This can be achieved through counter-storytelling, to enable Minoritised nurses and midwives to have space/s to share their experiences to enable anti-racism pro-action and challenge and disrupt the dominance of whiteness.

CRT's concept of the permanence of racism – the understanding that racial dynamics are deeply embedded in society and must be acknowledged to create meaningful change. This principle helps explain how White privilege manifests in nursing education. Such disparate treatment directly influences how Minoritised nurses and midwives develop their sense of belonging and worthiness in clinical environments. Through CRT's principle of the permanence of racism, we can understand how racism's entrenchment in society enables some White individuals to justify or normalise discriminatory behaviours. Moving forward requires White individuals to recognise and understand that their racialised identity inherently provides them with certain societal advantages, influence and benefits (Schroeder & DiAngelo, 2010; Van Herk et al., 2011).

Critique of liberalism in nursing, while seemingly well-intentioned, as seen in interpretations of the NMC Code of Conduct (NMC, 2018a) means that White individuals do not always recognise the barriers experienced by Minoritised people. This denial can ultimately prevent meaningful policy changes needed to address social inequities.

This is supported by nurses and midwives' perception of the Nursing and Midwifery Council (NMC) Code of Conduct (NMC, 2018a), where patients are "treated equally" and therefore this ideology is carried over into the nursing workforce. However, claiming that you cannot see the skin colour of individuals perpetuates racism, and the message received is that individuals do not recognise the daily barriers, exclusions and structural advantages that exist for Minoritised people (McGibbon et al., 2014; Thorne, 2017). Therefore, this allows society to ignore legislation or policies that enhance social inequalities and inequities.

The application of CRT's tenet of interest convergence highlights that policies to address racialised equality are aimed at benefiting White people. Concerningly, the NMC is problematic in itself. The NMC (2024a) independent culture review, found that the NMC is a toxic, racist and bullying workplace and because of this, their fitness to practice investigations are impacted – "In the course of our review we heard of many poor behaviours including racism, bullying and discrimination. But while these combined to create a toxic culture in certain parts of the organisation, it begged the question: how have these deep-seated issues ultimately impacted on the NMC's mission to protect the public?" (NMCl, 2024a, p. 16).

The NMC's (2024a) independent culture review revealed systemic issues of racism. The NMC, which oversees both registered and student nurses and midwives, must ensure its organisational behaviour, leadership, policies and guidelines actively combat racism and protect staff who report concerns. A milestone outcome for Equality 4 Black Nurses (2025), a legal principle, was identified, as the tribunal found that the NMC "the body entrusted with protecting public safety, can itself be a vehicle of racial retaliation. When wielded to punish rather than protect, a referral may constitute unlawful victimisation under the Equality Act 2010."

Nurses and midwives are deemed to be at the forefront of advocacy and ensuring equality as specified in the NMC Code of Conduct (NMC, 2018a). However, structural racism within nursing, and its regulatory body, still exists, and this requires dismantling (Broome & Villarruel, 2020). Advocating for social justice is a responsibility of the nursing profession, and professional body, as outlined in the NMC Code of Conduct (NMC, 2018a). This is supported by CRT, which encourages White people to use their power and privilege to dismantle oppressive structures.

CRT has a strong desire towards social justice to change the world for the better. The main target is to dismantle oppressive systems (Airhihenbuwa & Ford, 2010). Critical race theorists look to transform and improve the world rather than observe only (Matsuda, 1991). This is achieved through research that leads to the foregrounding of racialisation and empowers underrepresented groups through equity and liberation (Solórzano & Yosso, 2001).

Using counter-narratives, within CRT can give Minoritised people and communities a voice and also demonstrate to others that they are encountering similar racial experiences.

CRT foregrounds counter-narratives because race is not normally discussed, and those who are affected by racism, and Minoritised suffer in silence, blame themselves, or act like the incident never happened (Delgado & Stefancic, 2017). Two case studies of racism will now be reviewed through CRT to demonstrate the entrenched racism in nursing and midwifery.

Erica's Story

The nursing profession, whilst championing values of care, compassion and equality, remains embedded within broader societal structures that perpetuate racial inequalities. This case study examines the experiences of Erica (name changed for confidentiality) a Black British nursing student, who encountered microaggressions during her clinical placement. Through the theoretical framework of CRT, this analysis explores how seemingly subtle interactions can reinforce systemic racism within healthcare education and practice. The review of Erica's story employs counter-narrative methodology to centre her voice and challenge dominant narratives that often marginalise the experiences of Black nursing students.

Erica, a 22-year-old second-year nursing student of Jamaican heritage, was undertaking a nursing placement as part of her course. Having excelled academically, she approached her placement with enthusiasm and confidence. The ward, a busy 30-bed unit, was staffed predominantly by White nurses, with Erica being one of only two Black students on placement during this period.

During her third week of placement, Erica was assigned to work with a Staff Nurse, a racialised White woman in her early 50s with 15 years of nursing experience. The morning began routinely with handover and initial patient assessments. However, as they approached the bed of a patient, an elderly White patient with diabetes, the dynamic shifted significantly.

The patient, upon seeing Erica, immediately turned to the Staff Nurse and stated, "I don't want her touching me. Can't you do it instead?" Staff Nurse paused momentarily before responding, "Don't worry, Erica is still learning. I'll handle your care today, and she can observe." Erica felt her stomach drop as she was relegated to the role of passive observer, despite having successfully performed similar procedures throughout her placement.

Later that morning, during the coffee break, the Staff Nurse approached Erica privately. "Don't take it personally, love," she said with what appeared to be genuine concern. "Some of the older patients are just set in their ways. It's nothing to do with you – they're just more comfortable with familiar faces. You'll understand when you've been qualified longer."

Erica's Counter-Narrative to the Story

When the patient rejected her care, Erica felt that familiar knot in her stomach from traumatic experiences that she had hoped she had left behind after secondary school. But what hurt more was watching the Staff Nurse immediately accommodate the request without question. In that moment, she was not seen as a competent nursing student who had successfully cared for dozens of patients – she was reduced to her racialised identity negatively.

The explanation about "older patients being set in their ways" felt like a betrayal to Erica. It suggested that racism was acceptable, that she should accept racialised discrimination as an inevitable part of her professional journey. When the Staff

Nurse told her not to take it "personally,' Erica wondered how something so fundamental about her identity as a Black woman could be anything but personal.

What frustrated Erica most was the lost learning opportunity. She had prepared thoroughly for that procedure, and suddenly she was relegated to watching from the sidelines. How many similar opportunities would she lose? How would this impact her clinical competence and confidence?

The incident made Erica question whether she truly belonged in nursing. If patients could simply refuse her care based on her race, and if qualified nurses would enable this behaviour, what kind of career was she entering? She felt isolated and began to doubt her abilities, despite her strong academic performance.

Critical Race Theory Analysis of Erica's Story

CRT recognises that race is a social construct used to maintain power hierarchies (Delgado & Stefancic, 2017). Counter-narrative methodology is central to CRT scholarship, providing space for marginalised voices to challenge dominant narratives (Delgado, 1995). Erica's account disrupts several problematic narratives commonly found in nursing education. Erica's experience illustrates how racial categories become salient in healthcare interactions, with her professional identity as CRT posits that racism is permanent and endemic to society. In Erica's case, the microaggression she experienced reflects deeper systemic issues within healthcare. The patient's overt racial preference and the nurse's accommodation of this preference demonstrate how racism is normalised and institutionalised within healthcare settings.

The concept of interest convergence suggests that progress and good change for racialised people occurs only when it serves White interests. The nurse's response exemplifies this principle – by framing the incident as protecting both the patient's comfort and Erica's feelings, she prioritises institutional harmony over challenging racism. Thus, relegating racism as being less important to upholding negative colonial ideas of people not racialised as White.

Dominant narratives in nursing often emphasise colour-blindness, suggesting that good nurses treat all patients equally regardless of racial background or heritage. Erica's experience reveals how this narrative obscures ongoing racial dynamics and prevents meaningful engagement with racism.

Nursing education frequently emphasises individual resilience and the need for students to adapt to challenging situations. Erica's counter-narrative highlights how this expectation places the burden of managing racism on its victims rather than addressing systemic issues. Nursing culture often demands professional neutrality and emotional regulation. Erica's account demonstrates how this expectation can silence discussions about racism and marginalise students' legitimate concerns.

Sue et al. (2007, p. 271) define racial microaggressions as "brief and commonplace daily verbal, behavioural, or environmental indignities, whether intentional or unintentional, that communicate hostile, derogatory, or negative racial slights and insults toward people of colour." The incident involving Erica encompasses multiple forms of microaggression:

> The patient's explicit refusal of care constitutes a micro assault – a deliberate discriminatory action. Whilst the patient's behaviour might be dismissed as individual prejudice, CRT analysis reveals how such incidents are enabled by systemic structures that prioritise patient preference over equity.
>
> The Staff Nurse's response represents a microinsult through its subtle derogation of Erica's professional capacity. By immediately agreeing to the patient's demand and positioning Erica as "still learning," she reinforced racial hierarchies while maintaining plausible deniability.
>
> The explanation that older patients are "set in their ways" serves as a microinvalidation, nullifying Erica's legitimate concerns about racial discrimination by reframing the incident as generational difference rather than racism.

The story has profound implications for Erica's learning and development. Research demonstrates that exposure to racialised microaggressions can negatively impact academic performance, mental health and professional identity development among students of colour (Sue et al., 2007), due to the mental cognitive overload that these experiences cause. The lost learning opportunity represents not merely an individual setback but a systemic barrier to fair, equitable and liberatory nursing education.

Nursing and midwifery education involves complex processes of professional socialisation through which students learn professional values, behaviours and identities. Erica's experience illustrates how these processes can reinforce racial hierarchies, potentially leading to the reproduction of discriminatory and harassing practices within the profession.

The mentor nurse's response reveals institutional complicity in maintaining racism and racial hierarchies. By normalising patient racial preferences, thus racism, and failing to challenge discriminatory behaviour, healthcare institutions perpetuate systemic racism whilst maintaining facades of equality, justness, inclusion and belonging.

Erica's experience represents far more than an isolated incident of patient preference. Her voice, centred in this analysis, challenges nursing, ergo midwifery, education to confront uncomfortable truths about racism whilst pointing toward more equitable futures. Her experience serves as both a cautionary tale and a call to action for educators, practitioners and institutions committed to justice in nursing education and practice. Through CRT analysis, it becomes clear that her encounter with microaggression reflects endemic racism within nursing education and healthcare practice. The counter-narrative methodology reveals how dominant discourses in nursing can marginalise and silence the experiences of Black students, perpetuating systemic inequalities and inequities. Only through honest engagement with

CRT principles and genuine commitment to anti-racist practice can nursing education and the profession begin to fulfil its stated values of justice, equality, inclusion and belonging.

Reviewing Racism in Tribunal Cases through Critical Whiteness Analysis

Critical whiteness scholarly activity and research is increasing, but CRT is better known and established. Critical whiteness is the study of how the White lies of superiority continues the status quo of racism in the system; that those who are racialised as White or align with White people believe they are superior humans, intellectually, culturally and in knowledge generation, are ambitious, hard-working and deserving of all opportunities above others to advance them in life (Gillborn, 2024; Mills, 2007; Parkin & Johnson, 2024). Gillborn (2024) asserts that even now, in current times, people racialised as White/White people are aggressively emboldened to legitimise racism and the primacy of White people's interests, while attempting to keep the latter in place by closing down on any critical viewpoint/s that opposes their claims of superiority and righteousness. Matias et al. (2014) summarises critical whiteness as studying how White people respond to Black reality(ies), hence critical whiteness studies support CRT by deconstructing White imaginings.

In this chapter in introducing this construct, critical whiteness is used to identify and analyse how whiteness manifests and its consequences for racialised people in the system, who are not White identifying, through reviewing two tribunal cases involving Black nurses.

Adelaide's Case

The first is of Adelaide Kweyama, a Black agency nurse who was racially abused by patients and the poor response of the manager when she raised her concerns to the situation (Gov.UK, 2023a; Salisbury, 2023). The recounting of the complaint is taken from the public record of the tribunal (Gov.UK, 2023c) and the reporting of the case in the Evening Standard online (Salisbury, 2023). While working for the National Health Service (NHS), in one incident, January 2019, Adelaide was confronted with racist comments, including the n-word, from a patient waiting for medication. The month following this incident there was more racial abuse from another patient. She reported these incidents to her then manager, another nurse. The comment that came back from the manager was that Adelaide needed to bathe in a pool of bleach so that it would whiten her skin, then apparently the patients would be more pleasant to Adelaide. The following day to this comment, she overheard the same nurse saying the same bleach comment to another nurse adding that she was fed up with nurses saying they were sick when at work. Adelaide submitted a complaint through the trust electronic process, but there wasn't any follow up due process to her complaint. When Adelaide had told the agency that the incidents were affecting her mental health causing depression, she was later told by the NHS manager that they were concerned about Adelaide's mental health from the content of her complaint. The tribunal's judgement of the case upheld the bleach comment as racial harassment and the raising of the mental health concern as victimisation (Gov.UK, 2023c).

So let's unpick this from a critical whiteness perspective.

Racist slurs from patients

Usually in NHS organisations you find there is a zero tolerance to abuse and violence of staff policy and campaign for patients and service users, but not zero tolerance for racism (BRAP & Kline, 2024). This aligns to whiteness not seeing racism as a necessary or real concern (Daniels, 1997). The NHS is majority people racialised as white, 74.6% (WRES, 2024), and this is somewhat mirrored in nursing and midwifery, reporting that 66% of their registrants identified as white out of 841,367 (NMC, 2024b). With a majority white population it is more likely that their voices are heard, their concerns given more attention, their culture is built into the system hence giving them an advantage, moreover racism is usually placed in the 'too hard to deal with box', hence racism is normalised and ignored (BRAP & Kline, 2024).

Whitening skin colour comment from manager

Colourism is a colonial construct that privileges those, especially directed at women, who are white or have lighter skin tone to be seen as more visually better, worthy of health, wealth and other life/living opportunities, also honest and having integrity (Spratt, 2023). By the comment to Adelaide about whitening her skin, the person making the comment is asserting that they are better and in power, or more powerful, this is the strategy of whiteness in the system to maintain the status quo of hierarchy based on colourism. Hence indicating that Adelaide is seen as lesser within the system.

Olukemi's Case

The next tribunal case is of Black midwife Olukemi Akinmeji, she successfully sued her employing trust "for discrimination and victimisation" upheld by the tribunal. "She faced a 'toxic' work environment in which her colleagues "ganged up" on her" (Gov.uk, 2023b, cited in BRAP & Kline, 2024, p. 30). From the tribunal judgement and feedback document (Gov.uk, 2023b):

On her last day, a senior colleague said that they should check Olukemi's bag because there had been thefts in the workplace.

When Olukemi finally made the complaint, there was a slowness of response, then misdirection by saying that the perpetrator had attended unconscious bias training due to the complaint, but this was false.

The tribunal found that another perpetrator had intent to malign Olukemi, e.g. calling out Olukemi on not using an instrument correctly in front of the patient or forbidding her to answer patients' buzzers.

The tribunal also found some actions and behaviour by lead staff were race motivated, these staff were White, e.g. not allowing Olukemi to leave early for a family matter when a lead staff was able to, not looked after when feeling unwell when a White staff was, a White staff getting longer breaks then Black and Brown staff.

Let's analyse Olukemi's case from a critical whiteness perspective.

Creating a white workplace environment

There were three lead staff who were white who asserted their power and whiteness status by creating difference in how they treated staff who were not racialised as white and white staff, e.g., comparatively white staff getting longer breaks and white staff looked after when unwell. In addition, these staff were trying to create a negative narrative around Olukemi, e.g. implying she was stealing and not competent regarding accusing her of not using the equipment correctly. These actions are creating an environment where all are not welcome to work, but those racialised as white are unconditionally welcome. In Adelaide's tribunal the judge summarised the consequences of a poor work environment, hence indicating the importance of a good working environment: "An environment is a state of affairs. It may be created by an incident, but the effects are of longer duration. Words spoken must be seen in context; that context includes other words spoken and the general run of affairs within the office or staffroom concerned" (Gov.UK, 2023c). Mills (1997) suggests that it is white ignorance at play, this is not passive but active operationalisation of controlling of Black and brown bodies/lives to keep the status quo practice of racism in the system.

Workplace slowness to respond to Olukemi's complaint

Much like Adelaide's case in this case the action of slowness and deflection, shows that racism is of little concern so there is no urgency to follow the complaint protocol (BRAP & Kline, 2024). Hence whiteness or white ignorance not 'seeing' racism as a necessary or real concern (Daniels, 1997) continuing to uphold racism in the system (Mills, 1997).

By viewing the cases through critical whiteness, it reveals the power dynamics at play to maintain racism in the system. It also supports that leadership, culture, policies and practices maintain the racialised hierarchy, with White at the top claiming it has the rights to life opportunities first. The analysis helps to understand what the manifestation of whiteness in the workplace is. By sharing the analysis, it arms all to see whiteness and find ways to disrupt or challenge it. By exposing whiteness in play helps to disrupt or interrupt its power in the system. To be able to act within the system, the workplace must be psychologically safe, meaning teams in organisations feel safe to be open, to oppose/disagree, to be creative and innovative without any negative recourse, leading to a work environment culture that welcomes all (Edmondson, 2019). This leads to better decision making and enable a culture of continuous improvement, healthy environment. Psychological safety, means that within teams in organisations they have permission for candour without any negative recourse, leading to motivated teams, better decision making and enable a culture of continuous improvement, healthy environment to be able to fail forward (Edmondson, 2019), that is able to fail forward in its actions to disrupt/interrupt the pull of whiteness in the system.

However there are limitations to critical whiteness studies in that it is centring that White people are the solution for racism. Blaisdell and Taylor Bullock (2023) suggest to disrupt this centring of whiteness, critical whiteness studies must stay aligned to the tenets of CRT, and build its actions on the knowledge shared by racialised peoples that are not White, to keep power and privilege of whiteness in check. Furthermore, some caution in that critical whiteness studies is not to be thought of as a panacea for White folk to fully engage in deeper change in attitudes and behaviours for racial justice (Christiani & Britt, 2024). But critical whiteness studies do give direction towards collaborating with racially minoritised groups with White folks' conceptualisations of anti-racism and solidarity to then push forward equitable, just and liberatory change for all. Anti-racism change has to be systemically driven and strategised for sustainability and impact.

Conclusion

The chapter introduces the topic of CRT and CWS and how to analyse racism in the system through case studies learning and applying these constructs. Critically reviewing cases of racism, whiteness oppression and discrimination applying these constructs is radical and helps with sense-making to find collaborative impactful actions towards sustainable anti-racism change. Hence moving away from performative, piecemeal or traditional actions that continue the status quo. Learning from such analysis approaches will disrupt the repeating data of racism in the system through informing to apply targeted (based on racialised data) and universal (based on encompassing the widest possible difference) actions for change. Embedding such critically anti-racism conscious approaches must not be a one-off reactionary process but an ongoing commitment to review, reimagine and reconstruct institutional leadership, policies, practices, education and training with accountability measures.

Recommendations for Practice

Healthcare institutions must implement comprehensive cultural responsiveness training for all staff that addresses both explicit bias and microaggressions. This training should be mandatory and annually updated with annual developmental objectives. Nursing and midwifery services to start the process of anti-racism have to reconstruct policy, practice, processes, leadership, culture, education and training must reconstruct with a universal design to be culturally responsive and take mission-critical approach to anti-racism strategy. Black and minoritised nursing students require additional mentorship support that acknowledges the unique challenges they face. Mentor training should include specific guidance on recognising and addressing racialised microaggressions. This will open up opportunities that education and training alone could not offer. Clear policies addressing patients' racialised preferences for treatment care and chaperoning must be developed consistently and implemented inline with evidence-base, not due to racism, this has to be transparent and nuanced. These policies should prioritise equity whilst managing complex clinical situations compassionately. Accessible and confidential reporting mechanisms for racial incidents must be established, with clear processes for investigation and resolution.

Reflective Activity

Having read the chapter, we invite you to reflect on your key learning and its implications for your professional practice as a nurse or midwife using Bain et al.'s (2002) 5R framework (p. 13–15):

- Reporting – What is it in your situation you want to transform after reading this chapter?
- Responding – What are your personal observations regarding your own situation/context in relation to what is raised in this chapter?
- Relating – What is/are the theoretical/research/data/legislative, etc., understandings relationship to under consideration in this chapter that you could apply to your situation/context?
- Reasoning – Identify how the chapter findings matter to your situation/context and how will you interrogate your situation/context and what will help you from this chapter.
- Reconstructing – Identify your action plans to reframe and rebuild a transformative way forward to change from the situation in your context.

References

Airhihenbuwa, C.O., & Ford, C.L. (2010). Critical Race Theory, race equity, and public health: Toward anti-racism praxis. *American Journal of Public Health, 100*(Suppl 1), S30–S35. https://doi.org/10.2105/AJPH.2009.171058

Bain, J.D., Ballantyne, R., Mills, C., & Lester, N.C. (2002). *Reflecting on practice: Students teachers' perspectives*. Post Pressed.

Bell, D.A. Jr. (1980). Brown v. Board of Education and the interest-convergence dilemma. *Harvard Law Review*, 518–533. https://doi.org/10.2307/1340546

Bennett, C., Hamilton, E.K., & Rochani, H. (2019). Exploring race in nursing: Teaching nursing students about racial inequality using the historical lens. *OJIN: The Online Journal of Issues in Nursing, 24*(2). https://doi.org/10.3912/OJIN.Vol24No02PPT20

Blaisdell, B., & Taylor Bullock, R. (2023). White imagination, Black reality: Recentering critical race theory in critical whiteness studies. *International Journal of Qualitative Studies in Education, 36*(8), 1450–1458. https://doi.org/10.1080/09518398.2022.2025484

Broome, M.E., & Villarruel, A.M. (2020). Beyond the naming: Institutional racism in nursing. *American Academy of Nursing, Nursing Outlook, 68*, 375–376. https://doi.org/10.1016/j.outlook.2020.06.009

Browne, G., Haydon, G., & Van der Riet, P. (2018). Narrative inquiry as a research methodology exploring person-centred care in nursing. *Collegian, 25*(1), 125–129. https://doi.org/10.1016/j.colegn.2017.03.001

Christiani, L., & Britt, L. (2024). White privilege, white grievance, and the limitations of white anti-racism. *Politics, Groups, and Identities, 12*(3), 700–721. https://doi.org/10.1080/21565503.2023.2224779

Daniels, J. (1997). *White lies: Race, class, gender and sexuality in white supremacy discourse*. Routledge.

Decuir, J., & Dixson, A. (2004). "So, when it comes out, they aren't as surprised that it is there": Using critical race theory as a tool of analysis of race and racism in education. *Educational Researcher, 33*, 26–31. https://doi.org/10.3102/0013189X033005026

Delgado, R. (1995). *Critical race theory: The cutting edge*. Temple University Press.

Delgado, R., & Stefancic, J. (2017). *Critical race theory*. New York University Press.

Demathews, D.E., & Watson, T.N. (2020). *No critical race theory isn't 'anti-American.' Education Week*. https://www.edweek.org/leadership/opinion-no-critical-race-theory-isnt-anti-american/2020/10

Edmondson, A.C. (2019). *The fearless organisation: Creating psychological safety in the workplace for learning, innovation and growth*. John Wiley & Sons.

Equality 4 Black Nurses (E4BN). (2025). *When an NMC Referral is Triggered not by Risk, but by Race. Landmark Legal Victory by E4BN.* https://www.equality4blacknurses.com/post/when-an-nmc-referral-is-triggered-not-by-risk-but-by-race-landmark-legal-victory-by-e4bn

Gillborn, D. (2015). "The Monsterisation of Race Equality: How Hate Became Honourable." In C. Alexander, J. Arday & D. Weekes-Bernard (Eds.), *The runnymede school report race, education, and inequality in contemporary Britain*. Runnymede Trust (pp. 6–9).

Gillborn, D. (2024). *White lies: Racism, education and critical race theory*. Routledge.

Gov.UK (2023a). *'Ms A Z Kweyama v Central and North West London NHS Foundation Trust' (2023) Watford Tribunal Hearing Centre, case 3319570/2019*. GOV.UK. https://www.gov.uk/employment-tribunal-decisions/ms-a-z-kweyama-v-central-and-north-west-london-nhs-foundation-trust-3319570-slash-2019

Gov.UK (2023b). *'Ms O Akinmeji v East Kent University NHS Trust' (2023). Ashford Tribunal Hearing Centre, case 2303204/2020*. GOV.UKwww.gov.uk/employment-tribunal-decisions/ms-o-akinmeji-v-east-kent-university-nhs-trust-2303204-slash-2020

Gov.UK (2023c). *Ms A Z Kweyama v Central and North West London NHS Foundation Trust: 3319570/2019*. https://assets.publishing.service.gov.uk/media/63513413e90e0731af6467d1/Ms_A_Z_Kweyama_v_Central_and_North_West_London_NHS_Foundation_Trust_3319570.2019_FMH_Reserved_Judgment.pdf

Harris, C. (1993). Whiteness as a property. *Harvard Law Review, 106*(8), 1707–1791. https://doi.org/10.2307/1341787

Hiraldo, P. (2010). The role of critical race theory in higher education. *The Vermont Connection, 31*, 53–59.

BRAP and Kline, R. (2024). *Too hot to handle: Why cases of racism are not heard or acted upon*. BRAP. https://27aa994b-a128-4a85-b7e6-634fb830ed15.usrfiles.com/ugd/27aa99_9a9468c5e4da43288da375a17092d685.pdf

Ladson-Billings, G. (1998). Just what is critical race theory and what's it doing in a nice field like education? *International Journal of Qualitative Studies in Education, 11*(1), 7–24. https://doi.org/10.1080/095183998236863

Ladson-Billings, G. (2005). The evolving role of critical race theory in educational scholarships. *Race, Ethnicity and Education, 8*, 115–119. https://doi.org/10.1080/1361332052000341024

Ladson-Billings, G., & Tate, W. (1995). Toward a critical race theory analysis of education. *Teachers College Record, 97*(1), 47–68. https://doi.org/10.1177/016146819509700104

Matias, C.E., Mitchell Viesca, K., Garrison-Wade, D.F., Tandon, M., & Galindo, R. (2014). What is critical whiteness doing in our nice field like critical race theory?" applying CRT and CWS to understand the white imaginations of white teacher candidates. *Equity & Excellence in Education, Equity & Excellence in Education, 47*(3), 289–304. https://doi.org/10.1080/10665684.2014.933692

Matsuda, C. (1991). Voices of America: Accent, anti-discrimination law, and a jurisprudence for the last reconstruction. *Yale Law Journal, 100*, 1329–1407.

Matsuda, M., Lawrence, C., Delgado, R., & Crenshaw, K. (1993). *Words that wound critical race theory, assaultive speech and the first amendment*. Westview. https://doi.org/10.4324/9780429502941

McCoy, D.L. (2006). Entering the academy: Exploring the socialization experiences of African American male faculty. https://repository.lsu.edu/gradschool_dissertations/3297/

McGibbon, E., Mulaudzi, F.M., Didham, P., Barton, S., & Sochan, A. (2014). Toward decolonizing nursing: The colonization of nursing and strategies for increasing the counter-narrative. *Nursing Inquiry, 21*(3), 179–91. https://doi.org/10.1111/nin.12042

Mills, C.W. (1997). *The Racial contract*. Cornell University Press.

Mills, C.W. (2007). White Ignorance. In S. Sullivan & N. Tuana (Eds.), *Race and epistemologies of ignorance*. State university of New York press (pp. 11–38).

Nursing and Midwifery Council (NMC). (2018). *The Code. Professional standards of practice and behaviour for nurses, midwives, and nursing associates*. Nursing and Midwifery Council.

Nursing and Midwifery Council (NMC). (2024a). Independent culture review. https://www.nmc.org.uk/globalassets/sitedocuments/independent-reviews/2024/nmc-independent-culture-review-july-2024.pdf

Nursing and Midwifery Council (NMC). (2024b). *Registration data reports: September 2024 mid-year data report*. https://www.nmc.org.uk/about-us/reports-and-accounts/registration-statistics/#:~:text=Between%201%20April%20and%2031

Parkin, R.A., & Johnson, K.R. (2024). Interrogating whiteness: Critical reflections on occupational science scholarship and social responsibility. *Journal of Occupational Science*, 1–14. https://doi.org/10.1080/14427591.2024.2312996

Salisbury, J. (2023). *London nurse told to 'bleach skin' after racism complaints wins £25,000 payout*. Evening Standard. https://www.standard.co.uk/news/london/nurse-told-to-bleach-skin-after-racism-complaints-wins-25k-payout-b1064565.html

Schroeder, C., & DiAngelo, R. (2010). Addressing whiteness in Nursing education: The sociopolitical climate project at the University of Washington School of Nursing. *Advances in Nursing Science, 33*(3), 244–255. https://doi.org/10.1097/ANS.0b013e3181eb41cf

Solórzano, D.G. (1997). "Images and words that wound: Critical race theory, racial stereotyping and teacher education." *Teacher Education Quarterly 24*(3), 5–19. http://www.jstor.org/stable/23478088

Solórzano, D.G., & Solórzano, R. (1995). The Chicano educational experience: A proposed framework for effective schools in Chicano communities. *Educational Policy, 9*, 293–314.

Solórzano, D.G., & Yosso, T.J. (2001). Critical race and LatCrit theory and method: *Counter-storytelling. Qualitative Studies in Education, 14*(4), 471–495. https://doi.org/10.1080/09518390110063365

Solórzano, D.G., & Yosso, T.J. (2002). Critical race methodology: Counter-storytelling as an analytical framework for education research. *Qualitative Inquiry, 8*(1), 23–44. https://doi.org/10.1177/107780040200800103

Spratt, T.J.R. (2023). Understanding light-skin privilege in relation to anti-Black racism: Colourism, racism-induced stress and poor health outcomes amongst Black British women. *Ethnic and Racial Studies, 47*(10), 1941–1963. https://doi.org/10.1080/01419870.2023.2252880

Sue, D.W., Capodilupo, C.M., Torino, G.C., Bucceri, J.M., Holder, A.M.B., Nadal, K.L., & Esqulin, M. (2007). Racial microaggression in everyday life: Implications for clinical practice. *American Psychologist, 62*(4), 271–286. https://doi.org/10.1037/0003-066X.62.4.271

Symenuk, P.M., Tisdale, D., Bearskin, D.H.B., & Munro, T. (2020). In search of the Truth: Uncovering nursing's involvement in colonial harms and assimilative policies five years post Truth and Reconciliation Commission. *Witness: The Canadian Journal of Critical Nursing Discourse, 2*(1), 84–96. https://doi.org/10.25071/2291-5796.51

Thorne, S. (2017). Isn't it high time we talked openly about racism? *Nursing Inquiry, 24*(4), 1–2. https://doi.org/10.1111/nin.12219

Van Herk, K., Smith, D., & Andrew, C. (2011). Examining our privileges and oppressions: Incorporating an intersectionality paradigm into nursing. *Nursing Inquiry, 18*(1), 29–39. https://doi.org/10.1111/j.1440-1800.2011.00539.x

Workforce Race Equality Standards (WRES). (2024). *NHS workforce race equality standards: 2023 data analysis report for NHS trusts*. NHS England. https://www.england.nhs.uk/long-read/workforce-race-equality-standard-2023-data-analysis-report-for-nhs-trusts/

3

ANTI-RACISM LEADERSHIP

Mushtag Kahin and Musharrat J. Ahmed-Landeryou

Introduction

This chapter will look at anti-racist leadership for nursing and midwifery primarily from a UK context, which will be transferable to other global contexts. Anti-racist leadership is an understanding of the intersectionality of racism, power and privilege and how it affects their organisations' performances/metrics, their staff and the service users' experiences. It also requires a commitment to change institutions from the core. Anti-racist leaders reflect on their biases and are committed to learning, even if it is a fail-forward context, within a safe and equitable environment to enable the organisation and all stakeholders to thrive (Evans, 2025).

The National Health Service (NHS) was created on 5 July 1948, allowing free healthcare to all, funded by taxpayers. The NHS could not have existed without the Windrush nurses, midwives and doctors from the West Indies. Almost 77 years later, the NHS is still institutionally racist as staff from the Global Majority continue to fare worse when it comes to discrimination, promotion, bullying, inappropriate referrals to regulatory bodies and raising concerns (Kapadia *et al.*, 2022; Kline, 2014; Kline, 2024). Furthermore, the NHS is institutionally racist towards patients too (Bamrah *et al.*, 2025) and is continuously not upholding its NHS constitution value that everyone counts. The NHS cannot exist without the workforce from the Global Majority and relies heavily on them to continue delivering its services (Kahin and Khan, 2023).

Many staff and patients from around the globe receive worse care and treatment from colleagues and professionals (BRAP and Kline, 2024; Kline, 2024). A few significant examples to highlight the disparities in healthcare are:

- Black pregnant women in the UK are four times more likely to die in healthcare (Felker and Knight, 2024).

DOI: 10.4324/9781003565369-3

- Black people are 3.5 times more likely to be sectioned under the UK Mental Health Act 1983 (amended in 2007) (GOV.UK, 2024).
- Black men are seven times more likely to endure police restraint (Inquest, 2023; NHS Digital, 2024).
- People who have Sickle Cell disease continue to receive poor care and are at risk of dying due to racial prejudice and a lack of knowledge from professionals (Delgado, 2025; NHS Race and Health Observatory, 2025).
- "Black nurses and midwives, as well as those of Unknown ethnicity, are disproportionately represented in the population of referrals to the NMC [Nursing and Midwifery Council – regulator in the UK]. Having qualified in Africa, as opposed to other continents, is also a risk factor for referral" (West *et al.*, 2017, p. 2).

Diversity and representation alone do not address the inequalities and inequities in the NHS or social care services, even with continuous evaluation, psychological safety, inclusion and sponsorship from top down (Sherbin and Rashid, 2017). When some Global Majority people make it to the top, they do not lift as they rise other Global Majority peers. Instead, it appears they mimic behaviours and actions that are emboldened through institutional racism; they do not want to lose and jeopardise what they have worked hard for, if not double or triple hard, compared to their racialised White colleagues, or those who align with whiteness. It is acknowledged that leaders from the Global Majority who are in very senior management Band 9 or Executive level, more than half have considered leaving the NHS due to racism (NHS Confederation, 2022). They themselves still feel precarious in their senior roles, hence their reluctance to be explicit in their actions to "lift as they rise". The majoritarian White groups in nursing and midwifery uphold discriminatory behaviours and actions due to multiple factors: leadership, policies, practices and cultures (BRAP and Kline 2024). These uphold institutional racism, whilst individuals blindly claim they themselves are not racist through failing to acknowledge their own whiteness, White privilege and culture of silence (DiAngelo, 2018; Iheduru-Anderson *et al.*, 2021; Schroeder and DiAngelo, 2010). Silence is complicity in keeping the status quo, a clear positional stance.

Anti-Racism Leadership

The Global Majority of nursing and midwifery staff have played a major role in nursing throughout history; however, we tend to celebrate white nursing figures, e.g. Florence Nightingale, who did not found nursing. The earliest Muslim nurse was Rufayda Al-Aslamiya, who introduced nursing to the world 1200 years before Florence Nightingale, which people do not know in general (Jan, 1996; Miller-Rosser *et al.*, 2006). Jewish nurse Emma Goldman was an anti-racist nurse, writer, philosopher and activist for social justice to reduce women's health inequalities (Women in Medicine Legacy Foundation, 2020). Harriet Tubman was a Black nurse and an anti-racist. She saved more people through nursing than through helping people escape slavery in the nineteenth century (Singleton, 2019).

Anti-racism and transcultural leadership are leadership approaches that take a systems approach to change, and to lead diverse staffing and embed inclusive, safer workplaces. It is paramount in the health and social care services to have leadership committed to this change and role-modelling anti-racist behaviour. Anti-racism leadership is fundamental to dismantling the systems' entrenched embrace of whiteness as the default. Whiteness centres those in the system who identify as racialised as White, or align to whiteness, as right, superior, civilised, trusted, affording opportunities and other privileges, whilst others are seen as lesser and less deserving (DiAngelo, 2018; Iheduru-Anderson *et al.*, 2021; Schroeder and DiAngelo, 2010). This status quo in the system is also continued due to internalised racism from some of the Global Majority staff and patients due to a lifetime of oppression, harm and embodied insecurity (Gooden and O'Doherty, 2015; Welton *et al.*, 2018).

Embedding anti-racism leadership provides better diversity and representation at higher levels (Williams and Mihaylo, 2019), which inspires hope in people from the Global Majority, because you cannot aspire to be what you never see. The McKinsey & Company report 2023 "Diversity Matters Even More" identifies that diverse teams with effective leadership lead to better staff satisfaction, creativity and opportunities and outperform organisations that do not support staff diversity by 39% (McKinsey and Company, 2023). This report is making a case for anti-racism leadership to drive culture change. In health and social care, anti-racism in nursing provides better culturally responsive patient care and prevents death while developing diverse leaders, reducing staff sickness and increasing staff satisfaction (Mostafa *et al.*, 2025). When staff members have equal access to career progression, Continuing Professional Development (CPD) and funded postgraduate training, they are more likely to feel valued as they have better opportunities to progress and develop into management and leadership. Anti-racist nursing and midwifery leadership should, in theory, drive a decrease in staff turnover through psychological safety, increase representation from top down and reduce the number of tribunals for racism, as accountability and justice will be taken by anti-racist leaders (Singh *et al.*, 2013).

Two Cases of the Consequences of Poor Leadership and Leadership Failure – Institutional Racism

Anti-Black racism towards Black nurses in the United Kingdom (UK) is situated in the system, as they are at higher risk of being referred by their employers, with eventually no case to answer at the regulatory body, the Nursing and Midwifery Council (NMC), after being hauled through this unnecessarily stressful process. However, White nurses are more likely to be referred by the public (West *et al.*,

2017). Within all this it is concerning that the NMC has been found to be institutionally racist as an organisation, perpetuating anti-Black racism, Islamophobia, bullying, lack of representation, ableism and staff having to work in a toxic environment and hence not living up to its values (Rise Associates and Afzal, 2024) Racial humility, accountability, commitment, evaluation and reflection are essential to dismantle anti-Black racism through transformative action (Massaquoi, 2023). However, it needs leadership from the regulator who is on board to direct the professional authentically from an equitable and justice-based accountability position, away from institutional racism.

In the USA, an award-winning Black nurse, DonQuenick Joppy, was compensated $20 million following unfair dismissal by her employer in retaliation after she raised discrimination in a landmark case (Book, 2025) – a case of anti-Black racism and the noxious consequences. DonQuenick Joppy was not promoted like her White peers, falsely accused by a White nurse, then investigated due to the false allegation, and put on a performance plan, which is a standard playbook found in healthcare for staff from the Global Majority. She was charged with manslaughter, which was later dropped, and Joppy became homeless, and her reputation and career were ruined. However, she fought back and won a civil rights lawsuit against HCA HealthOne Medical Center of Aurora. The court decided on the 19 of August 2025, unanimously "that Joppy's termination was the result of both retaliation for her complaint about race discrimination and race discrimination itself" (Book, 2025). This is in line with BRAP and Kline's (2024) study, which states that the person raising the concern of racism is victimised and made into the perpetrator by the organisation. But Joppy's final vindication was at a cost to her personal, social, psychological and financial well-being. Anti-racism is a lifelong process of unlearning, learning, continued reflection and intentional proaction for change in the system. In Joppy's case, this was not carried out due to institutional racism upheld by leadership and boards embracing whiteness.

Joppy's disturbing case occurred because racism is enabled in the health and social care organisations, because whiteness is in play in the system, enabled by leadership and facilitating cultures. "White tears", a term meaning, a psychological and emotional manipulation by a person racialised as White when they feel their privilege and status are being threatened by a person of colour (Hamad, 2021), giving precedence over reality and facts to the detriment of the Global Majority staff and patients. Usually, in these cases, Human Resources can be weaponised as a tool of oppression and harm to remove the person from the organisation. An issue here could be the lack of regulation of NHS management and Human Resources, hence resulting in delayed accountability, as in Joppy's case. When regulatory bodies are institutionally racist, such as the NMC (Rise Associates and Afzal, 2024) and the General Medical Council (GMC) (Razai, 2021), it enables institutional racism to continue where health and social care staff work.

In another landmark case, NHS England has been found guilty of racism and spent a substantial amount of public money on a case against a senior Black nurse leader, Michelle Cox (Ms A Cox v NHS Commissioning Board, (GOV.UK, 2023)). Ms Cox, a registered nurse of 25 years and an NHS continuing care manager, blew the whistle on poor practice and racial discrimination by her White manager. Due to this, she was treated with hostility and racism and excluded by a White manager, Gill Paxton, from any discussions regarding job opportunities for promotion. Initially, Ms Cox took her grievance to her organisation, and NHS England rejected it (Evans, 2023). Not satisfied with how the investigation into her grievance was carried out, Ms Cox took her case to the tribunal and won. The tribunal found that "Ms Paxton – who is now an associate director of nursing in the West Yorkshire integrated care system – had created an 'intimidating and hostile and humiliating environment' for Ms Cox, which had the purpose and effect of unlawful harassment. The tribunal also upheld Ms Cox's complaint of detriment for whistleblowing" (Kituno, 2023). In this situation, Ms Cox was faced with a White woman's tears, which comes from discomfort, fragility and the superior positioning of whiteness when it comes to having the power to cause or create racialised distress and harm (DiAngelo, 2011; Hamad, 2021; Phipps, 2021).

Moreover, we have White CEOs making anti-racism their brand; however, the data from actions in their organisations speak differently regarding the impact of anti-racism change (NHS England, 2025; BRAP and Kline, 2024). Hence, anti-racism and transcultural leadership in the health and social care sector from the top down is paramount for the psychological safety of staff and patients to speak up and out without fear of persecution and contribute to good change. We need anti-racism actions in strategy, and leaders and boards should be held accountable by sector regulators if they do not deliver.

Hindrances to Embedding Anti-Racism Leadership

Leadership holds the culture (Cote, 2023). Anti-racism embedding and culture change cannot happen without leaders and boards committing to and role modelling anti-racism (Kline, 2020). If they do not learn and unlearn, do not lean into introspection and discomfort from doing the anti-racism change, bring Global Majority stakeholders to the table to codesign and coproduce, the change they seek will not be authentic and will be transient. Disrupting whiteness in the system is a cultural change, not a "band-aid" type move or quick win. These latter two lead to a transient change. Leaders are constantly pushed to make change and show outcomes quickly, but to show anti-racism change in the metrics will take a couple of years, plus, this is change management 101. Pushing for quick change leads to gaming and engagement disingenuity of the anti-racism process, because boards and leaders are facing to meet the metrics instead of facing the staff, and hence patients, to improve their experiences and improve their opportunities. Government and boards always overestimate the abilities of leaders to make quick change (Janke *et al.*, 2020).

The system does not hold leaders accountable for anti-racism work. Leaders seem to move on to better jobs, or stay in their current jobs, even if they have poor performances in the NHS. Anderson (2012) says the problem is the boards, and puts forward three issues:

- *Like Protects Like:* The people on the boards are of similar backgrounds, hence they want to protect their own. Especially as leaders in the NHS are still a White men's boys club clique.
- *Hope Springs Eternal:* The board is in hope always that the leader or CEO did a good thing once and continually waits for the return of good outcomes from the leadership of the person. This is probably linked back to "like protects like" in the hope that his person will come good again.
- *Stick to the Tried and True:* Boards are living in the past. NHS leaders and boards are probably older people who have been in the business a while and continue to use the same solutions that worked for them in the past, even though how the world ticks are different. Again, back to "like protects like".

The WRES (Work Race Equality Standards) 2024 identify the limited diversity at leadership and senior executive levels (NHS England, 2025). This lack of diversity leads to a lack of diversity of thought, creativity, innovation and decision-making to improve organisation performance in regard to anti-racism (McKinsey and Company, 2023; Spillett, 2024). Evidence shows that organisations that support diversity have teams that excel (Carucci, 2024). Diverse teams have better innovative working and retaining talents (Hengartner, 2024). Having diverse leadership does not automatically translate to being anti-racist. Anti-racism is not only an active and lifelong commitment to unlearn and relearn about different cultures, religions and protected characteristics, but also changing the cultural status quo through organisational policies, practices and processes, i.e. in your organisation, there is education on being anti-ableist, and policies are written to support the disabled worker and students. This should be similar for anti-racism. The intersection of discriminations of anti-Blackness, islamophobia, antisemitism, neurodiversity, ableism, caste and class discrimination, and more, has many different harms and effects for people and communities. This is intersectionality, when our different identities come together to disadvantage us. It was originally developed by Kimberlé Crenshaw (1989, 1991) in relation to systemic and institutional racism in the law. Organisational leadership does not seem to be cognisant of intersectionality and understand how it could disrupt the status quo for a just and sustainable anti-racism strategy.

The culture has a strong pull to enable whiteness in the system. Hence, leaders and senior executives who are usually racialised White are not held to account and therefore, are enabled to continue with poor anti-racism outcomes and institutional racism without accountability. When NHS Trusts' leaders, executives and managers are not held accountable by boards through key performance indicators by funding or regulation, they are able to keep on in their current job or move on to another NHS Trust with impunity, a continuing system failure.

What Leaders Have to Do to Be Impactfully Anti-Racist and Deliver Sustainable Anti-Racism Organisations

Anti-racism leaders have to take a systems approach to their work, because racism is embedded in the system. Spillett (2024) applies an anti-racism lens to the four themes of effective systems change by Bigland *et al.* (2020):

1. *Getting Started*

Put out a call to action to gather co-conspirators, a coalition of people across stakeholder groups, to codesign and coproduce effectively towards a common anti-racism purpose. Understand the system not only through quantitative data but also through qualitative data. The latter, in terms of deep narratives to gauge the multiple components of racism, to then start planning solutions to implement. Think also about how you share your findings effectively and efficiently. Everyone holds each other accountable, especially the leader.

2. *Making Momentum*

A key element of systems leadership is maintaining and sustaining anti-racism change effectively.

a) Structures

Governance – Lay out for all stakeholders the anti-racism governance structure, that is, the rules, practices and processes that ensure quality decision-making. A governance framework, also known as a governance structure, is essential for guiding how organisations operate and interact with stakeholders. It establishes the rules, practices and processes that dictate how decisions are made and who is accountable for those decisions. The primary purpose of a governance framework is to ensure that organisations operate in a legal, ethical and sustainable manner, ultimately benefiting all stakeholders involved and holding leaders to account. To do this, there must be learning about the history of racism and how racism is enabled in systems.

Resources – To the anti-racism work, there must be resources, monetary, human and material. This must be dedicated to the strategy; otherwise, importance will not be given to the work.

b) Cultures

Anti-racism work is relational work and is healing because it is nurturing by removing harm. Leaders need to build strong, effective relationships with stakeholders, to value their time, involvement, expertise and commitment to join in the anti-racism work. These co-conspirators will build resilience into the system so that it has the capacity and capability to adapt to the anti-racism change requirements.

c) People

Leaders need to build a community of learning that is safe and trusted, where open conversation, that debate and challenge are encouraged. The leaders are enabling the continued development of the coalition of co-conspirators and to lean into uncomfortable situations. Anti-racism leaders should show a wise, compassionate leadership approach in anti-racism work and initiatives. That is creating robust relationships to bring humanity and wisdom into the hard work of anti-racism, thus being an effective leader by being courageous, competent and truly taking care of people (Hougaard *et al.*, 2020).

3. *Paradoxes: Power, Conflict, Uncertainty*

a) Power

In systems leadership, you should map out where the power dynamics are and how to capitalise and remove/reduce the influence of those that hinder the anti-racism work. Anti-racism leaders should not only know their own power but also be open to sharing their power to advance the anti-racism agenda. Leads should be educated and educate regarding the strength of the interrelationship of power, racism and whiteness and plans on how to disrupt this relationship.

b) Conflict

Anti-racism leaders should lean into tension, debate and disagreement, as this will create space for further learning, challenge and manage conflict healthily through wise, compassionate leadership.

c) Uncertainty

Do not wait for perfection or having all the information, leaders should support action and use double loop learning, i.e. single loop learning is solving a problem, double loop learning is reviewing what the consequences of solving the problem are and acting further, and this is continuous (Argyris, 1976). Also, a fail-forward learning is encouraged.

4. *Indicators of Success*

a) A sense of enjoyment and a shared Endeavour

This work must align with the values and principles of anti-racism leadership, which align with the personal and professional values of people taking part. There must be equal Global Majority representation and diversity in the group doing the work to avoid groupthink. "Working together to improve racial equity in recruitment, retention and promotion to overcome the barriers of discrimination, racism and disparities will give a feeling of positive difference and progress. The NHS WRES and Social Care WRES are tools that can demonstrate positive changes to celebrate in their work" (Spillett, 2024, pp. 21). In Critical Race Theory (CRT), they would name it interest convergence, making the anti-racism work matter to the executives and organisation, because what matters gets attention.

b) Increased Momentum with Gains to the System

An indication of success is increased funding or more people joining in the work and increasing recognition of the work. This is all driven by leadership empowering people to do the anti-racism work for change.

c) Shifts in Evaluation Metrics

"A rebalancing of racial disparities and disproportionality that can be seen to be improving by a system that understands systemic racism and how to tackle it" (Spillett, 2024, pp. 21). You have to have both quantitative and qualitative data to measure the work.

Silent leadership in the NHS means complicity. We need to start naming and shaming them until real accountability is created. Why are those with the most power and decision-making not regulated and have the freedom to move around after failures and harm? We need WRES data linked to funding, CQC, KPIs and leadership. It has to start from the top down, and NHS England, not having any diversity in the Executive Board, is not leading by example and action. We need regulatory bodies like the NMC and GMC to be diverse in boards and panels, change their screening criteria to be anti-racist and train and review their staff competencies in anti-racism and cultural competence every year. This should also be mandatory for NHS staff, especially at induction and Personal Development Review. Led by a team of WRES experts, EDI leads, anti-racism experts, legal experts, HR experts, lived experience experts and anti-racist health and social care managers and leaders, they could provide advice for the first instance for staff or employers. Staff tend to leave bad leadership, not their work.

Audre Lorde (1993, pp. 94) once said, "The master's tools will never dismantle the master's house". This is exactly what anti-racism leadership is tackling, doing radically different using different for the benefit of all.

Conclusion

Anti-racism leadership is a personal commitment and reflection of a person's integrity and values. Recruiting authentic, culturally responsive and emotionally intelligent leaders with a proven track record of delivering anti-racism actions as a part of the solution in dismantling systemic racism in the NHS. Increasing representation helps inspire staff from the Global Majority to become leaders and improve their qualities. Diverse leaders should be enabled to create further diversity in leadership; however, policies, regulations and external bodies that monitor effectively are necessary. Anti-racism is a lifelong process, and this is why it is paramount for all staff working in the health and social care sector to have mandatory training by experts. This includes annual performance objectives to keep up with anti-racism practices and service delivery, as well as their personal development in the area. NHS Trust senior management should share learning from Tribunals with their staff and have a reflective practice in addressing anti-racism. Antiracist leadership empowers people to do the right thing by role-modelling and proactively demonstrating their credibility so that they can be trusted by staff from the Global Majority to create an equitable, just and safe working environment.

We need brave (future) leaders and managers who are comfortable being uncomfortable and have insights into how systemic racism, especially anti-Blackness, nepotism, discrimination and sexism affect the NHS workforce and culture. Only then can leaders authentically begin the urgent change of anti-racism.

Reflective Activity

Having read the chapter, we invite you to reflect on your key learning and its implications for your professional practice as a nurse or midwife using Bain *et al.*'s (2002) 5R framework (pp. 13–15):

- Reporting – What is it in your situation you want to transform after reading this chapter?
- Responding – What are your personal observations regarding your own situation/context in relation to what is raised in this chapter?
- Relating – What is/are the theoretical/research/data/legislative etc understandings relationship to under consideration in this chapter that you could apply to your situation/context?
- Reasoning – Identify how the chapter findings matter to your situation/context and how will you interrogate your situation/context and what will help you from this chapter?
- Reconstructing – Identify your action plans to reframe and rebuild a transformative way forward to change from the situation in your context.

References

Rise Associates and Afzal, N. (2024). *The Nursing and Midwifery Council Independent Culture Review*. https://www.nmc.org.uk/globalassets/sitedocuments/independent-reviews/2024/nmc-independent-culture-review-july-2024.pdf

Anderson, E. (2012). Why Bad CEOs Get to Keep Their Jobs. *Forbes*, 18 May. https://www.forbes.com/sites/erikaandersen/2012/05/18/why-bad-ceos-get-to-keep-their-jobs/

Argyris, C. (1976). Single-loop and double-loop models in research on decision making. *Administrative Science Quarterly, 21*(3), 363–375. https://doi.org/10.2307/2391848

Bain, J.D., Ballantyne, R., Mills, C. and Lester, N.C. (2002). Reflecting on Practice: Students Teachers' Perspectives. Post Pressed.

Bamrah, J.S., Womersley, K., Nagpaul, C., Coghill, Y., Issa, R. and Hazard, L. (2025). NHS must tackle racism and sexism for the benefit of patients, staff, and society. *BMJ*, 390m https://doi.org/10.1136/bmj.r1334

Bigland, C., Evans, D., Bolden, R. and Rae, M. (2020). Systems leadership in practice: Thematic insights from three public health case studies. *BMC Public Health, 20*(1), 1–14. https://bmcpublichealth.biomedcentral.com/articles/10.1186/s12889-020-09641-1

Book, C. (2025). Jury Awards Nurse DonQuenick Joppy $20M for Discrimination Lawsuit. *Nurse Org*. https://nurse.org/articles/nurse-donquenick-joppy-case/

Carucci, R. (2024). *One More Time: Why Diversity Leads to Better Team Performance*. https://www.forbes.com/sites/roncarucci/2024/01/24/one-more-time-why-diversity-leads-to-better-team-performance/

Cote, C. (2023). How Does Leadership Influence Organisational Culture? *Harvard Business School Online*, 2 March. https://online.hbs.edu/blog/post/organizational-culture-and-leadership

Crenshaw, K. (1991). Women of color at the center: Selections from the third national conference on women of color and the law: Mapping the margins: Intersectionality, identity politics, and violence against women of color. *Stanford Law Review, 43*(6), 1241–1279 https://doi.org/10.2307/1229039

Crenshaw, K.W. (1989). Demarginalizing the Intersection of Race and Sex: A Black Feminist Critique of Antidiscrimination Doctrine, Feminist Theory and Anti-Racist Politics. *University of Chicago Legal Forum* (pp. 139–67).

Delgado, C. (2025). Are patients with sickle cell disease still being failed by the healthcare system? *BMJ, 390*. https://doi.org/10.1136/bmj.r847

DiAngelo, R. (2011). White fragility. *International Journal of Critical Pedagogy, 3*(3), 54–70.

DiAngelo, R. (2018). White Fragility. Why It Is So Hard for White People to Talk About Racism. Beacon Press books.

Evans, N. (2023). Racism in the NHS: Could landmark ruling on discrimination be a watershed moment? *Nursing Management, 30*(3), 7–9. 10.7748/nm.30.3.7.s2

Evans, N. (2025). *Anti-Racist Leadership: Why It Matters and How to become One*. https://www.embracingequity.org/post/anti-racist-leadership-why-it-matters-and-how-to-become-one#:~:text=Anti-racist%20leadership%20is%20understanding%20your%20how%20your%20racial,environment%2C%20and%20supporting%20people%20through%20equitable%20organizational%20structures

Felker, A. and Knight, M. (2024). *Saving lives, improving mothers' care: Lessons learned to inform maternity care from the UK and Ireland Confidential Enquiries into Maternal Deaths and Morbidity 2020–22*. https://www.npeu.ox.ac.uk/assets/downloads/mbrrace-uk/reports/maternal-report-2024/MBRRACE-UK%20Maternal%20MAIN%20Report%202024%20V2.0%20ONLINE.pdf

Gooden, M.A. and O'Doherty, A. (2015). Do you see what I see? Fostering aspiring leaders' racial awareness. *Urban Education, 50*(2), 225–255. https://doi.org/10.1177/0042085914534273

GOV.UK. (2023). Manchester Employment Tribunals, Ms A Cox v NHS Commissioning Board 2415350/2020 + 24 1365/20 1. https://www.gov.uk/employment-tribunal-decisions/ms-a-cox-v-nhs-commissioning-board-operating-as-nhs-england-slash-nhs-improvement-2415350-slash-2020-and-2401365-slash-2021

GOV.UK. (2024). *Detentions Under the Mental Health Act.* https://www.ethnicity-facts-figures.service.gov.uk/health/mental-health/detentions-under-the-mental-health-act/latest/#main-facts-and-figures

Hamad, R. (2021). White Tears, Brown Scars. Melbourne University Press.

Hengartner, D. (2024). *The Power of Diversity in Innovation Teams.* https://www.forbes.com/councils/forbesbusinesscouncil/2024/10/24/the-power-of-diversity-in-innovation-teams/

Hougaard, R., Carter, J. and Hobson, N. (2020). Compassionate Leadership Is Sufficient – but Not Enough. *Harvard Business Review.* https://www.harvardbusiness.org/wp-content/uploads/2021/02/HBR_2020_12_compassionate-leadership-is-necessary-but-not-sufficient.pdf

Iheduru-Anderson, K., Shingles, R.R. and Akanegbu, C. (2021). Discourse of race and racism in nursing: An integrative review of literature. *Public Health Nursing, 38*(1), 115–130. https://doi.org/10.1111/phn.12828

Inquest (2023). *New report: Black men seven times more likely to die following police restraint but racism not being addressed.* https://www.inquest.org.uk/police-racism-report-2023

Jan, R. (1996). Rufaida al-Asalmiya, the first Muslim nurse. *The Journal of Nursing Scholarship, 28*(3), 267–268. https://d1wqtxts1xzle7.cloudfront.net/96853111/j.1547-5069.1996.tb00362.x20230105-1-3l0e59-libre.pdf?1672919509=&response-content-disposition=inline%3B+filename%3DRufaida_Al_Asalmiya_the_First_Muslim_Nur.pdf&Expires=1757102878&Signature=DvU3J3vXC4-bP9eO7-L8anhXHNAZXvRkDNE6vL-n99JmbBcsuJL2T8PVes1QFhTV6SJgobOeQ1F~AuH6ywy3A97z~n25nUoSwNJv5GIu6E6eyFjEiAMBCiaSUbHZxIijEvVn~oTP6Sl7UuUAL683ZOBJhO8PCe6qMxtOPwZ4NgJFole2EPfLgWzoWY-sFmZnQazF9Xwxdm8Dh1aX8qNlleT8nbpecb-3Mz3Nbx5hL1oRUTaBCs9aYjxH46xpd6qz9HZGrdnmhPN8PExmdcUvKYnug2wv-Qfz8VY1yHNn1KImp4mto~449v4Nb6Sn0acKzPMmzn~FpAgZYknlyehMfnA__&Key-Pair-Id=APKAJLOHF5GGSLRBV4ZA

Janke, K., Propper, C. and Sadun, R. (2020). The impact of CEOs in the public sector: Evidence from the English NHS. *Harvard Business School.* https://scholar.harvard.edu/files/rsadun/files/the_impact_of_ceos_in_the_public_sector-_evidence_from_the_english_nhs.pdf

Kahin, M. and Khan, N. (2023). Healthcare inequalities and social justice blog series: Transcultural leadership, anti-racism, and psychological safety. *BMJ Leader.* https://blogs.bmj.com/bmjleader/2023/10/18/transcultural-leadership-anti-racism-and-psychological-safety-by-by-mushtag-kahin-and-dr-nagina-khan/

Kapadia, D., Zhang, J., Salway, S., Nazroo, J., Booth, A., Villarroel-Williams, N., Bécares, L. and Esmail, Aneez, A. (2022). Ethnic Inequalities in Healthcare: A Rapid Evidence Review. NHS Race and Health Observatory. https://nhsrho.org/research/ethnic-inequalities-in-healthcare-a-rapid-evidence-review-3/

Kituno, N. (2023). NHSE wrongly dismissed discrimination claim from black nurse, tribunal finds. *Health Service Journal (HSJ).* NHSE wrongly dismissed discrimination claim from black nurse, tribunal finds | News | Health Service Journal

Kline, R. (2014). The Snowy White Peaks of the NHS: A survey of discrimination in governance and leadership and the potential impact on patient care in London and England. *Middlesex University Research Depository.* http://eprints.mdx.ac.uk/13201/

Kline, R. (2020). After the speeches: What now for NHS staff racial discrimination? *BMJ Leader.* https://blogs.bmj.com/bmjleader/2020/06/13/after-the-speeches-what-now-for-nhs-staff-race-discrimination-by-roger-kline/

BRAP and Kline, R. (2024). *Too hot to handle? Why concerns about racism are not heard or acted on.* https://27aa994b-a128-4a85-b7e6-634fb830ed15.usrfiles.com/ugd/27aa99_4d4e620e6889408d926dad142839c0f3.pdf

Kline, R. (2024). *Ten years on: The Snowy White Peaks of the NHS. BMJ Leader.* https://doi.org/10.1136/leader-2024-001022

Lorde, A. (1993). *The master's tools will never dismantle the master's house*. In C. Moraga and G. Anzakdia (eds.), This Bridge Called My Back: Writings by Radical Women of Colour. Kitchen Table Press (pp. 94–101).

Massaquoi, N. (2023). Racial humility over competence: Addressing anti-Black racism and healthcare leadership responsibility. *Healthcare Management Forum, 36*(5), 280–284. https://doi.org/10.1177/08404704231186807

McKinsey and Company. (2023). *Diversity matters even more: The case for holistic impact*. https://www.mckinsey.com/featured-insights/diversity-and-inclusion/diversity-matters-even-more-the-case-for-holistic-impact

Miller-Rosser, K., Chapman, Y. and Francis, K. (2006). Historical, cultural, and contemporary influences on the status of women in nursing in Saudi Arabia. *Online Journal of Issues in Nursing, 11*(3). https://doi.org/10.3912/OJIN.Vol11No03PPT02

Mostafa, I., Onwumere, J. and Wood, L. (2025). A systematic review and thematic synthesis of healthcare professionals' experiences of racism in the workplace and the support they receive. *Journal of Workplace Behavioral Health*, 1–29. https://doi.org/10.1080/15555240.2025.2519298

NHS Confederation. (2022). *Shattered hopes: Black and minority ethnic leaders' experiences of breaking the glass ceiling in the NHS*. https://www.nhsbmenetwork.org.uk/wp-content/uploads/2022/06/Shattered-hopes-1.pdf

NHS Digital. (2024). *Detentions under the Mental Health Act*. https://www.ethnicity-facts-figures.service.gov.uk/health/mental-health/detentions-under-the-mental-health-act/latest/

NHS England. (2025). *Workforce Race Equality Standard: 2024 data analysis report for NHS trusts*. https://www.england.nhs.uk/publication/nhs-workforce-race-equality-standard-2024-data-analysis-report-for-nhs-trusts/

NHS Race and Health Observatory. (2025). *Sickle cell comparative review to inform policy report*. https://nhsrho.org/wp-content/uploads/2025/06/SICKLE-CELL-COMPARATIVE-REPORT-.pdf

Phipps, A. (2021). White tears, white rage: Victimhood and (as) violence in mainstream feminism. *European Journal of Cultural Studies, 2*(1), 81–93. https://doi.org/10.1177/1367549420985852

Razai, M.S. (2021). Racism at the GMC—It is time to take action. *The BMJ Opinion*. https://blogs.bmj.com/bmj/2021/07/15/racism-at-the-gmc-it-is-time-to-take-action/

Schroeder, C. and DiAngelo, R. (2010). Addressing whiteness in Nursing education: The sociopolitical climate project at the University of Washington School of Nursing. *Advances in Nursing Science, 33*(3), 244–255. https://doi.org/10.1097/ANS.0b013e3181eb41cf

Sherbin, L. and Rashid, R. (2017). Diversity doesn't stick without inclusion. *Harvard Business Review*, 1–5. https://www.harvardbusiness.org/wp-content/uploads/2020/07/HBR-Diversity-Doesnt-Stick-Without-Inclusion.pdf

Singh, B., Winkel, D.E. and Selvarajan, T.T. (2013). Managing diversity at work: Does psychological safety hold the key to racial differences in employee performance? *Journal of Occupational and Organizational Psychology, 86*(2), 242–263. https://doi.org/10.1111/joop.12015

Singleton, M. (2019). *Flashback Friday—Harriet Tubman's Overlooked Story as a Nurse*. https://nursing.virginia.edu/news/flashback-harriet-tubman-nurse/

Spillett, M. (2024). *Anti-racist systems leadership to address systemic racism. Research In Practice*. https://www.researchinpractice.org.uk/media/sooflams/anti-racist-practice-strategic-briefing-joint_web.pdf

Welton, A., Diem, S. and Carpenter, B.W. (2018). Negotiating the politics of anti-racist leadership: The challenges of leading under the predominance of Whiteness. *Urban Education, 54*(5), 627–630. https://doi.org/10.1177/0042085918783830

West, E., Nayar, S., Taskila, T. and Al-Haboubi, M. (2017). *The progress and outcomes of Black and Minority Ethnic (BME) nurses and midwives through the Nursing and*

Midwifery Council's Fitness to Practice Process. https://www.nmc.org.uk/globalassets/sitedocuments/other-publications/bme-nurses--midwives-ftp-research-report.pdf
Williams, J.C. and Mihaylo, S. (2019). How the best bosses interrupt bias on their teams. *Harvard Business Review, 97*(6), 151–155. https://hbr.org/2019/11/how-the-best-bosses-interrupt-bias-on-their-teams
Women in Medicine Legacy Foundation. (2020). *Radicalization of a Nurse: The Story of Emma Goldman.* https://www.wimlf.org/blog/radicalization-of-a-nurse-the-story-of-emma-goldman

4

ANTI-RACISM IN NURSING AND MIDWIFERY EDUCATION

A Pathway to Social Justice

Joel Wunimasim Daanyaya, Miranda Leach, and Precious Adade Duodu

Introduction

Racism remains a deeply entrenched issue in healthcare, nursing and midwifery education. The COVID-19 pandemic further spotlighted long standing health inequities that have deep-seated roots in structural racism (Canadian Association of Schools of Nursing (CASN), 2023; Davis et al., 2024). Nursing students from Global Majority backgrounds continue to experience racism and discrimination in clinical placements (Caffrey et al., 2023; Dafny et al., 2025; Walker et al., 2023) and in universities (Bell, 2021; Hantke et al., 2022; Playfair et al., 2023). As a profession that has its fundamental principles rooted in social justice through the promotion of human dignity, equity in care and non-maleficence, the failure to address racism is making the nursing profession and its training grounds "toxic and unsafe environments" that can undermine professional development (Caffrey et al., 2023, p. 1). Even more concerning is the findings of a recent independent culture review into the Nursing and Midwifery Council (NMC) UK; one of the largest healthcare regulators in the world, which concluded that the NMC is institutionally racist (NMC, 2024). This reinforces the need to critically interrogate not only individual bias, but also structural and institutional forms of racism embedded in nursing and midwifery.

As the most trusted and largest group of health professionals, the International Council of Nurses (ICN, 2023) argues that nurses are in a powerful position to dismantle the structures that perpetuate racialised inequality and racism. The values that underpin professional nursing practice have their roots in social justice; thus, nurses have a professional and moral duty to act to challenge racial injustice (Boakye et al., 2024; Mello, 2023). Social justice is concerned with the fair treatment of all people advanced through the principles of equity, access, participation

DOI: 10.4324/9781003565369-4

and human rights (American Association of Colleges of Nursing (AACN), 2021a). Yet, despite the general acceptance of the need for the promotion of social justice and decades of research on the negative impact of racism on health outcomes, the pivotal role of nurse educators in advancing anti-racism in nursing education is underdeveloped and lacks a consistent and evidence-based guidance. This chapter argues that the future of nursing and midwifery education requires a paradigm that leads to a transformational shift from passive awareness of racism to being actively anti-racist. This shifting is the moving away from rhetorical commitments to diversity, towards actively embedding anti-racist praxis across curricula, pedagogy, assessment and institutional structures. Thus, the role of nurse educators and the nursing education system is crucial in shaping curricula and learning experiences that produces nurses and midwives who are competent and confident in tackling racism in all its forms. Taken together, cultivating a socially just and anti-racist nursing workforce begins with education. This chapter thus draws on the literature on anti-racist research and practice in nursing and midwifery and provides nurse educators with actionable strategies aimed at equipping future nurses with the competence, courage and confidence to be anti-racist in every context of care.

Setting the Scene: Anti-Racism Nursing and Midwifery Education

A recent definition by the American Nurses Association (ANA) describes racism as: "assaults on the human spirit in the form of actions, biases, prejudices, and an ideology of superiority based on race that persistently causes moral suffering and physical harm of individuals and perpetuates systemic injustices and inequities" (ANA, 2022). This definition implicates both individual and systemic levels of racism. As stated by Kishimoto (2018), when racism is only understood as individual prejudice, racism embedded at the institutional level is overlooked. At the individual level, there is significant evidence that highlights its deleterious impact on those who experience it (Bheenuck et al., 2007; Burnett et al., 2020; Krieger, 2014; McChesney, 2015). Persistent exposure to the stress of the experience of racism adversely affects body systems causing diseases such as hypertension and diabetes (Boakye et al., 2024), premature labour and low birthweight (Playfair et al., 2023) and other significant health conditions. As Williams et al. (2019) strongly asserts, the evidence unequivocally demonstrates that racism has detrimental effects on all aspects of a person's life.

Traditional nursing and midwifery curricula are situated in dominant structures of White, Eurocentric perspectives (Bell, 2021). Furthermore, nursing and midwifery is dominated by whiteness (Iheduru-Anderson & Waite, 2022) and the standardisation of whiteness signifies norm, privilege and dominance. Tracing the sociohistorical roots of nursing and midwifery curricula reveals how it has been framed through a White lens and whiteness seen as the default and other cultures as deviations or deficiencies. As Puzan (2003) argues, the centrality of whiteness in nursing and midwifery education normalises and reproduces systemic

White privilege which continues to disadvantage non-White students and by extension, patients. This foundational position of nursing and midwifery makes race ignorance possible and fails to bring to the fore the impact of racism as the root cause of inequities and disparities in health. Key stakeholders such as nursing and midwifery educators play a crucial role in either reinforcing or dismantling these structures. When educators are more concerned about preserving harmony and homogeneity in order not to experience the discomfort of challenging racism (Burnett et al., 2020), their actions and inactions further reinforce racism (Playfair et al., 2023). This lack of commitment by the relevant stakeholders coupled with an inconsistent and clear conceptual and methodological approach to anti-racism education has given rise to the criticism that nursing education is complicit in delivering "politically soft curricula" (Bell, 2021, p. 3). Politically soft curricula superficially acknowledge diversity and inclusion but does not tackle the roots of systematic racism that produces structural inequalities. This only perpetuates inequities and is akin to putting a band aid on a deep wound.

It has become undeniably evident that nursing education cannot continue the pretence of ignoring the impact of racism. Silence is not neutral and a sustainable anti-racist approach to nursing and midwifery education is needed now than ever before.

Towards Anti-Racism Nursing and Midwifery Education

Anti-racism is defined as an active process of identifying and eliminating racism through an intentional process of changing systems, attitudes, policies and practices that ensures the equitable redistribution of power (Davis et al., 2024). To address racism in nursing and midwifery education, there needs to be a shift from a passive position of "not being racist" to a more active role of being anti-racist (Verma, 2022). These ideas of transforming nursing and midwifery education through anti-racism are in tandem with the tenets of Critical Race Theory (CRT) which promotes activist pedagogy. CRT is discussed in detail in Chapter 2 of this book. CRT offers a powerful analytical lens which acknowledges that racism is a deeply embedded feature of society and supports anti-racist approaches that not only considers racism at the individual level but extends to dismantling the systemic roots of racism.

Indeed, Kendi (2019) argues that there is no neutrality in racism; one is either actively anti-racist or one is racist. Discourses on anti-racism highlight that whilst nurse educators do not deny racism, they are reluctant to address them head-on (Playfair et al., 2023). It is worth noting, however, that nursing stakeholders globally have shown some commitment to integrating anti-racism into nursing education, practice and research.

The Canadian Association of Schools of Nursing (CASN) published guidance aimed at promoting anti-racism nursing education in Canada which reinforces the urgency for critical anti-racist action in nursing education (CASN, 2023). The guidance which is situated in the context of diversity in Canada posits that nursing schools must create a culture of collective, institutional anti-racism and allyship in tackling racism. American nursing scholars have also proposed The Health Professions Anti-Racism Framework as a structured approach in integrating anti-racist principles into healthcare education (Davis et al., 2024). Their framework is birthed from the premise that a multidisciplinary approach is needed to develop comprehensive anti-racist curricula. It emphasises a curriculum that recognises the historical impact of race on health inequities and teaches students to be critical in their analysis of how race has been operating in the background. In the United Kingdom, the National Health Service (NHS) England, in partnership with the NHS Confederation and the NMC have produced a resource to support nursing and midwifery professionals in tackling racism (NHS England, 2022). These guidance, frameworks and resources indicate a bold ambition to achieve anti-racism. However, as Bell (2024) argues, the saying of anti-racism is not the doing of anti-racism. Whilst all these efforts are needed in promoting anti-racism, the systemic nature of racism means that a comprehensive process of sustainably embedding anti-racism through anti-racist nursing education is imperative. The following sections draw from the vast literature on anti-racism to suggest evidence-based, practical and actionable strategies in sustainably adopting an anti-racist approach in nursing education.

Component Features of Anti-Racist Nursing and Midwifery Education

The imperative to embed anti-racism within the fabric of nursing and midwifery education is no longer a peripheral concern but a central tenet for fostering health equity and upholding the ethical foundations of the profession. Anti-racist nursing and midwifery education moves fundamentally beyond earlier, often inadequate, approaches such as cultural competence or sensitivity, which frequently failed to address the structural roots of inequality and risked perpetuating stereotypes through a focus on cultural difference (Hantke et al., 2022; Playfair et al., 2023). Instead, anti-racism demands a proactive, intentional and ongoing commitment to identifying, analysing and dismantling the systems, ideologies and practices that perpetuate racial hierarchy and discrimination within healthcare and education itself. It is, Blanchet Garneau et al. (2023) articulate, a "learned, intentional, and strategic effort" aimed not merely at awareness but at tangible action and systemic transformation.

Nursing and midwifery, as professions entrusted with the health and well-being of all individuals, therefore bear profound ethical obligations, embedded within their professional standards, to confront and actively oppose racism not only as an interpersonal failing but as a structural determinant of health that poisons the healthcare system and contributes to these unjust outcomes. As such, achieving authentic anti-racist nursing and midwifery education requires a multifaceted approach, integrating several core components that work synergistically to challenge the status quo. This section explores the essential features, arguing that they represent the foundational pillars upon which effective and transformative anti-racist pedagogy must be built. These components include: cultivating critical consciousness and reflexivity amongst both educators and students; diversifying the curriculum to centre Black and Minoritised knowledge and explicitly address structural racism; implementing anti-racist pedagogical strategies that foster critical dialogue and challenge power dynamics; reimagining anti-racism approaches to assessment and evaluation to ensure equity; fostering institutional commitment to drive systemic change through monitoring and evaluating operationalising of allocated policy and resources and supporting faculty development and wellbeing to equip educators for this challenging but vital work. Each component is not discrete but crucial, and their interdependence necessitates a holistic and integrated strategy within nursing and midwifery education institutions. Any meaningful anti-racism educational transformation is a reviewing, reframing and rebuilding, starting with collaborating with Black and Minoritised students and spring-boarding pedagogical change from their voices.

Component 1: Cultivating Critical Consciousness and Reflexivity

A foundational component of any genuine commitment to anti-racist nursing and midwifery education lies in the deliberate cultivation of critical consciousness and reflexivity among both educators and learners. This involves moving beyond superficial awareness towards a deep, analytical understanding of how systems of power, privilege and oppression, particularly those rooted in race and whiteness, shape individual experiences, professional practices and health outcomes. As highlighted by Blanchet Garneau et al. (2023), developing a critical understanding of power relationships and moving towards critical consciousness are essential prerequisites for meaningful anti-racist action. It requires an uncomfortable but necessary interrogation of one's own positionality within these systems and recognising how these positions influence perspectives, interactions and clinical judgements. This means acknowledging how factors such as racial background/heritage, class, gender and other intersecting identities confer unearned advantages or disadvantages.

The process begins with fostering profound self-awareness regarding personal biases, assumptions and complicity in maintaining racist structures. This is not a one-off exercise but an ongoing, iterative practice. Hantke et al. (2022) emphasises the importance of confronting the ways whiteness operates, often invisibly, to uphold racial hierarchies, even though seemingly benevolent or neutral stances within nursing and midwifery. Educators, particularly those racialised as White, or aligning to whiteness, must critically examine how their own socialisation and professional training may have internalised dominant, often Eurocentric, norms and perspectives, potentially leading to the unwitting perpetuation of racism (Playfair et al., 2023). Similarly, students must be guided to explore their own backgrounds and biases, understanding how these might impact their interactions with patients, colleagues and the healthcare system.

Component 2: Diversifying the Curriculum

The nursing curriculum itself stands as a critical site for anti-racist intervention. Traditional nursing and midwifery education, often deeply rooted in Eurocentric perspectives and biomedical models, has historically Minoritised and marginalised or altogether excluded the knowledge, experiences and contributions of racialised communities, while simultaneously failing to adequately address the structural determinants of health inequities, particularly racism (Hantke et al., 2022; Suárez-Baquero, 2024). Therefore, a core component of anti-racist nursing and midwifery education involves the deliberate and thorough process of diversifying the curriculum. This requires moving beyond tokenistic additions towards a fundamental re-evaluation and foundational restructuring of what knowledge is valued, taught and assessed. It requires the incorporation of indigenous health knowledge and healing practices, foregrounding the theoretical contributions and research of scholars from racialised backgrounds, and including perspectives from the Global South to counter the dominance of Western viewpoints (Blanchet Garneau et al., 2023).

Representation within learning materials is also essential. We need to interrogate what knowledge is included and what is marginalised, made invisible or purposefully excluded. For example, why do we not refer to the original Blackfoot indigenous conceptualisation of hierarchy of needs where Maslow stayed with the Sisika Nation people and from their knowledge developed his Western version of hierarchy of needs (Bray, 2019). Case studies, clinical scenarios, imagery and assigned readings must reflect the diversity of the populations nurses and midwives serve and challenge stereotypical portrayals. Such representation comprises ensuring that the contributions of nurses, midwives and health leaders from diverse racial backgrounds are highlighted throughout the curriculum, not just in designated "diversity" modules. This curricular transformation becomes business-as-usual, fundamentally reconstructive, and necessary to create a learning environment where multiple ways of knowing are validated, and the complex realities of intersectional racism and health and care are confronted directly.

Component 3: Implementing Anti-Racist Pedagogical Strategies and Brave Spaces

Complementing a diversifying curriculum requires the adoption of pedagogical strategies that actively embody anti-racist principles. How content is taught is as crucial as what content is taught in fostering an environment conducive to critical learning about racialisation and racism. This component focuses on the teaching methods and classroom dynamics necessary to move beyond passive knowledge acquisition towards active engagement with anti-racist praxis. It implies the explicit move beyond outdated models of cultural competence or cultural humility towards a pedagogy grounded in anti-racism and structural competence to be culturally responsive and responsible. While cultural humility encourages self-reflection, anti-racist pedagogy demands a direct confrontation with power structures and systemic inequities (Hantke et al., 2022; Iheduru-Anderson & Waite, 2024; Playfair et al., 2023).

An anti-racism education in nursing and midwifery must have the characteristic of equipping students not just to interact respectfully with diverse individuals, but to recognise and challenge the racism embedded systems impacting their health and care (Iheduru-Anderson & Waite, 2024). Additionally, creating learning environments where candid, albeit challenging, conversations about race and racism can occur is paramount. Often termed "brave spaces", these environments prioritise mutual respect and accountability, encouraging participants to engage authentically with sensitive topics, acknowledge discomfort and learn from differing perspectives (Ford et al., 2024; Iheduru-Anderson & Waite, 2022). "Brave spaces" is related to the concept of psychological safety for individuals and groups in organisations and is created by leadership engendering an anti-racism cultural environment through strategising policies and practices which enable creativity, innovation and belonging (Edmonson, 2018). Facilitating such spaces requires significant skill from educators, including the ability to manage conflict, address microaggressions constructively and fairly and ensure that discussions remain focused on systemic issues rather than devolving into individual defensiveness or avoidance (Playfair et al., 2023). This contrasts sharply with traditional classroom dynamics where such topics might be avoided, delegitimised, devalued or superficially addressed.

Component 4: Reimagining Anti-Racism Assessment and Evaluation

It is impossible to discuss the components of anti-racism education in nursing and midwifery without mentioning assessment and evaluation. Traditional assessment methods (i.e., standardised testing, objective structured clinical examinations (OSCEs), quantitative measures) are not neutral; they can inadvertently perpetuate systemic biases and disadvantage students from Black, Minoritised and marginalised backgrounds (Coddington & Karsten, 2014; Sokolowich, 2025). Assumptions about objectivity can mask culturally specific communication styles, differing expressions of knowledge and the impact of stereotype threat on performance. Therefore, a key component of anti-racist nursing education involves critically examining existing assessment strategies and actively developing and implementing equitable alternatives that genuinely measure the desired competencies, including the application of anti-racist principles.

Universal Design for Learning (UDL) offers a transformative and forward-thinking framework for fostering equity in assessment. Rather than relying on reactive accommodations, UDL advocates for designing educational strategies from the outset to meet the needs of diverse learners. In nursing education, empirical evidence underscores the power of UDL to enhance accessibility, promote inclusivity and boost learner engagement through its core principles: multiple means of representation, action and expression (Scheirer, 2021; Kotcherlakota et al., 2024; Celestini & Palalas, 2024). Beyond nursing, broader educational research affirms these advantages, demonstrating that UDL effectively dismantles barriers and advances equity across varied learning contexts (Kavitha, 2023). Yet, despite its promise, implementation challenges persist. Nursing faculty frequently cite obstacles such as limited professional development, inadequate institutional support and the considerable time investment required to redesign assessments and curricula (Harris, 2018; Levey, 2018). From a wider higher education perspective, scholars caution that without careful alignment to professional and regulatory standards, UDL-inspired assessments risk becoming overly generalised, potentially undermining the measurement of specialised competencies (Abayasekara, 2021). Moreover, embedding UDL is not merely a pedagogical shift—it demands a cultural transformation. Institutions and educators must move from a reactive model of accommodation to a proactive model of equity (Anderson et al., 2019; Cressey, 2020).

Taken together, insights from nursing and broader educational scholarship position UDL as a compelling pathway towards more equitable assessment practices. However, its success hinges on sustained institutional commitment, robust faculty development and strategic alignment with professional standards—ensuring that inclusivity is achieved without compromising academic rigor.

The initial step requires a thorough audit of current assessment tools and practices to identify potential sources of racialised bias. This includes scrutinising the language and cultural assumptions embedded in exam questions and clinical scenarios, evaluating the diversity of assessors and simulated patients and considering how high-stakes, timed assessments might disproportionately affect students navigating linguistic barriers or systemic stressors. The existing literature suggests that reliance on supposedly objective measures can fail to capture crucial aspects of competence and demonstration of knowledge and understanding, such as critical thinking about health equity, effective cross-cultural communication and the ability to challenge systemic barriers (Blanchet Garneau et al., 2023). Thus, developing equitable, universally designed assessment strategies necessitates a move towards methods that value diverse ways of knowing, understanding and demonstrating competence. Specifically, assessments must explicitly evaluate students' understanding and application of anti-racist principles in both theoretical work and clinical practice. This could involve assessing their ability to identify racism in clinical scenarios, articulate strategies for intervention, demonstrate advocacy for racialised patients and reflect critically on their own role in perpetuating or challenging inequities.

Furthermore, programme evaluation itself must adopt an anti-racist lens. Evaluating the effectiveness of anti-racist initiatives within the nursing programme requires looking beyond simple student satisfaction surveys. It involves collecting and analysing data disaggregated by race to identify disparities in student progression, retention and achievement; assessing the impact of curricular changes on students' critical consciousness and practice; evaluating the institutional climate regarding race and inclusion; really, it is concerning measuring belonging and seeking meaningful feedback from students, faculty and community partners from racialised groups (Playfair et al., 2023).

Component 5: Fostering Institutional Commitment and Systemic Change

While curriculum reform, pedagogical innovation and critical consciousness are vital, their impact remains limited without a corresponding commitment to systemic change at the institutional level. It requires the full weight of the institution's leadership, resources and policies to dismantle entrenched structures that perpetuate inequity. As Playfair et al. (2023) assert, without institutional support, individual educators face insurmountable barriers in changing the pervasive culture of racism often found within educational and healthcare settings. Therefore, fostering genuine institutional commitment is an indispensable component of sustainable anti-racist transformation.

This commitment must begin with visible and unwavering support from institutional leadership. Deans, directors and senior administrators must champion anti-racism as a core strategic priority, allocating dedicated funding and resources for initiatives such as curriculum development, faculty training, student support services and robust data collection systems for monitoring equity outcomes. Rhetorical commitments are insufficient; tangible investment signals the institution's seriousness and provides the necessary infrastructure for change (Blanchet Garneau et al., 2023). This leadership buy-in is crucial for overcoming inertia and potential resistance within the institution.

Beyond resource allocation, institutional commitment manifests through the development and implementation of explicit anti-racist policies across all operational domains. Admission and recruitment processes for both students and faculty must be critically reviewed and redesigned to actively promote diversity and equity, moving beyond tokenism to address systemic barriers that disadvantage racialised applicants. Hiring, retention and promotion practices need similar scrutiny, ensuring that criteria value anti-racist scholarship and practice, and that mechanisms are in place to support and retain faculty from diverse backgrounds, particularly those engaged in challenging anti-racist work (Playfair et al., 2023).

Also, institutions must establish clear accountability mechanisms to track progress and ensure that anti-racist goals are met. Achieving this would mean setting measurable objectives, regularly collecting and transparently reporting data disaggregated by racialised groups (e.g., on admissions, progression, retention, faculty diversity, reported incidents of racism) and implementing robust systems for reporting and addressing allegations of racism experienced by students, staff or faculty (Iheduru-Anderson & Waite, 2022). In clinical rotations, students should be made aware of prevailing racial health disparities, since evidence shows that teaching about inequities in patient outcomes deepens understanding of social determinants of health and prepares students to deliver more equitable care (Davis et al., 2024; Williams et al., 2019).

Clinical preceptors play a pivotal role in shaping student experiences during placements, particularly when students encounter racism, which can lead to psychological distress and undermine their professional identity. Evidence shows that structured debriefing facilitated by trained preceptors can help students process these incidents, reduce harm and foster the development of anti-racist competencies (Dafny et al., 2025; Johnson et al., 2021; Walker et al., 2023). Scholars further advocate for equipping preceptors with the skills to engage in meaningful dialogue about racism, validate student experiences and model inclusive practice within clinical learning environments (Boakye et al., 2024; Crenshaw et al., 2025; Ford et al., 2024).

Component 6: Supporting Faculty Development and Wellbeing

The successful implementation of anti-racism nursing and midwifery education hinges significantly on the training, capacity, competence and wellbeing of the faculty tasked with delivering it. Many educators, particularly those socialised within predominantly whiteness embedded systems, may feel ill-prepared, resistant or unaware of their own biases and complicity in upholding racism structures (Hantke et al., 2022; Playfair et al., 2023). Therefore, robust and sustained faculty development, coupled with attention to wellbeing, constitutes a critical component of any institutional anti-racism strategy. Mandatory, comprehensive and ongoing anti-racism training for all faculty members is essential. This training must move beyond superficial diversity workshops towards deep engagement with CRT, whiteness studies, intersectionality and the history of racism in healthcare and education (Hantke et al., 2022), with yearly development through targeted appraisal objective setting for accountability and responsibility for operationalising anti-racism change. It should equip faculty with the knowledge to understand systemic racism and the skills to identify, challenge and create change within their own practice and the institution. Furthermore, specific training is needed to develop faculty knowledge, understanding and competence in facilitating difficult conversations about racism in the classroom, managing intersectional racialised conflict constructively and creating inclusive learning environments where students feel safe yet challenged to engage critically (Blanchet Garneau et al., 2023; Boakye et al., 2024).

Particular attention must be paid to the support and mentorship needs of faculty from racialised backgrounds who engage in anti-racism work. These faculty members often carry a disproportionate burden in leading anti-racism initiatives, educating colleagues and supporting students of colour, while potentially facing resistance, devaluing, delegitimisation, marginalisation or tokenism within the institution (Playfair et al., 2023). Institutions must actively foster supportive environments, as faculty of colour engaged in anti-racism work frequently encounter professional isolation, tokenism and the pressure of representing racialised perspectives within predominantly White academic spaces. Research underscores the value of structured support networks—such as affinity groups, cross-departmental collaborations and equity-focused councils—in offering safe spaces for shared experiences, reducing isolation and cultivating collective resilience (Ro et al., 2021; Hamilton & Haozous, 2017). Equally vital are mentorship opportunities that promote retention, professional development and wellbeing. Faculty of colour often lack access to informal mentoring networks that benefit their White counterparts, limiting their progression into leadership roles (Mkandawire-Valhmu et al., 2010). Formal mentorship programmes—especially those pairing junior faculty with culturally responsive senior mentors—can enhance scholarly output, build confidence and support career advancement (Ro & Villarreal, 2023; Akintade et al., 2025). These programmes should also address strategies for navigating systemic racism in academia. To ensure sustainability, institutions must embed mentorship and anti-racist efforts into formal structures, including recognition in workload models, promotion criteria and resource distribution. When such contributions are treated as invisible or supplementary, faculty of colour face increased risk of burnout and attrition. Institutionalising these efforts signals a genuine commitment to equity and inclusion (Hamilton & Haozous, 2017; Ro & Villarreal, 2023).

Although these six elements form the foundational pillars of anti-racist nursing and midwifery education, their enduring influence hinges on the institution's ability to maintain, embed and evolve them over time. The next section outlines approaches for integrating anti-racism into the structural and cultural fabric of nursing and midwifery education to support sustained transformation.

Making It Last: Sustainable Anti-Racist Education for Nursing and Midwifery

Anti-racist education in nursing and midwifery must move beyond reactive responses to social movements or accreditation pressures to become a sustained, adaptive and institutionally embedded commitment to equity. This requires shifting from episodic efforts to proactive, systemic strategies resilient to political cycles and leadership changes. Sustainability means not only ensuring the longevity of anti-racist initiatives but also enabling them to evolve with changing healthcare, societal dynamics and professional standards (Benner et al., 2010; Blanchet Garneau et al., 2023). To meet current and future healthcare demands, nursing and midwifery education must prioritise inclusive, culturally responsive training that prepares graduates to address persistent health disparities affecting Black and Minoritised communities (Betancourt et al., 2003; Boakye et al., 2024). Strategic planning should support ongoing programmes that embed adaptability and equity in academic and clinical contexts, producing clinicians who deliver ethical, evidence-based and justice-oriented care. Sustainability also requires anti-racist curricula that equip learners to recognise and disrupt systemic inequalities, improving patient outcomes and trust (Betancourt et al., 2003). Co-created professional development, grounded in anti-racist principles and designed with students and faculty, ensures education remains current, evidence-based and responsive to practice realities (Boakye et al., 2024). As the AACN (2009, 2021b) asserts, continuous education must dismantle discriminatory structures and cultivate inclusive learning spaces where equity is foundational rather than aspirational. This section therefore examines sustainable strategies for embedding anti-racism through governance, leadership accountability, faculty development, stakeholder engagement and continuous evaluation, drawing lessons from past initiatives to build inclusive and resilient systems.

1. Institutionalisation and Governance

For anti-racist nursing and midwifery education to be sustainable, it must be embedded within institutional structures so that anti-racism is not treated as temporary or dependent on individual champions, but as a core value shaping policy, accreditation, strategy and governance (Boatright et al., 2018; NLN, 2024). Key strategies include:

a ***Embedding equity into accreditation, quality assurance and curriculum revisions:*** Accrediting bodies such as AACN (2021b) and NLN (2024) require measurable progress in diversity, equity and inclusion. These standards must permeate curriculum design, faculty recruitment, student support and graduate competencies. Diversity cannot be confined to stand-alone modules but woven across all courses—from anatomy to ethics—to normalise equity in every aspect of training (Ackerman-Barger et al., 2020).

b ***Strategic planning and mission alignment:*** Institutions should explicitly prioritise anti-racism in their mission statements and strategic plans. This signals long-term commitment and provides a framework for resource allocation and accountability. Recruitment and retention strategies must deliberately target underrepresented student and faculty groups, ensuring equity is structurally supported rather than aspirational.

c ***Inclusive governance structures*:** Boards, committees and leadership teams must reflect the diversity of the communities they serve. Decision-making processes must include historically marginalised voices to prevent equity goals from being diluted or sidelined.

Institutionalisation shifts anti-racism from aspiration to accountability. Credibility depends on demonstrable equity outcomes (Ackerman-Barger et al., 2020), and without structural reform, diversity standards risk tokenism (Boatright et al., 2018). Sustained progress requires leaders to continually evaluate and reform policies, dismantling systemic barriers that undermine equity (IOM, 2011). Without such embedding, anti-racist initiatives remain performative rather than transformative.

2. *Mandatory Training, Accountability and Policy Alignment*

Anti-racism must be a systemic imperative, central to nursing and midwifery education. Sustainability requires mandatory, ongoing, evidence-based training for all roles—preceptors, faculty and students—focused not just on awareness but on cultivating critical consciousness of identity, bias and structural determinants of health (Ackerman-Barger et al., 2020; AACN, 2021a; Blanchet Garneau et al., 2023). Reflective journals, debriefs and discussions enable learners to process issues of race, power and privilege, while culturally affirming, psychologically safe environments with diverse case studies and simulations directly address bias and microaggressions (Jeffreys, 2015; Gonzalez et al., 2021; Moorley & West, 2022).

Sustainability further depends on leadership accountability—with senior leaders championing anti-racism, resourcing reform, publishing diversity metrics and responding decisively to discrimination (Boakye et al., 2024). Thus, long-term sustainability requires contemporary policies that enshrine equity goals, transparent accountability systems and leadership structures that prioritise anti-racism as central to educational quality (Boatright et al., 2018; Ackerman-Barger et al., 2020). Furthermore, policy alignment is essential. Admissions, assessment, placement and support systems must be critically reviewed to dismantle barriers and embed equity throughout the student journey (Ackerman-Barger et al., 2020; AACN, 2021a). Finally, research are key as further inquiry is needed into innovative pedagogies, the effectiveness of anti-racism training, and the long-term outcomes of justice-based education on reducing health disparities. This includes the development of accountability systems that evaluate not just diversity metrics but also the depth of structural change (Benner et al., 2010; Williams et al., 2019).

Together, training, accountability and policy reform establish anti-racism as a professional and organisational standard, not an optional project.

3. *Faculty Development and Wellbeing*

Faculty are central to anti-racist education: they shape learning environments, model professional behaviours and determine whether pedagogy is transformative or rhetorical. Development must be continuous, comprehensive and structurally embedded, as evidence shows sustained training improves teaching, outcomes and curricula (IOM, 2011; Benner et al., 2010).

Effective faculty development should include:

a ***Anti-racist pedagogy training:*** Equipping educators to teach racism, privilege, intersectionality and structural determinants of health, while facilitating difficult dialogues and modelling allyship. Training must go beyond superficial diversity sessions to include anti-racist pedagogy, implicit bias and cultural humility—embedded in appraisal and promotion for accountability (American Nurse Journal, 2024; Boakye et al., 2024). Faculty resistance, institutional inertia and student discomfort must be met with sustained faculty development, continuous training and reformed curricula that are consistently backed by leadership commitment (Day & Beard, 2019; NLN, 2024).

b ***Structural competence and cultural humility:*** Deepening understanding of systemic inequities (housing, employment, policy) and integrating them into teaching. Institutions must also hire, retain, and mentor diverse faculty, modelling inclusivity and disrupting whiteness in nursing education (Blanchet Garneau et al., 2023).

c ***Peer learning and reflective practice:*** Fostering communities of practice for shared reflection, innovation and accountability while reducing isolation (Hamilton & Haozous, 2017; Ro & Villarreal, 2023). Embedding case-based and practice-oriented learning or real-world case studies operationalising anti-racism strategies enable students to engage critically with health disparities, develop clinical judgment and apply equity principles in authentic scenarios (Jeffreys, 2015; Gonzalez et al., 2021).

Institutions must also address "cultural taxation", where racialised faculty disproportionately shoulder anti-racism work, leading to burnout and attrition. Valuing this labour in workload, tenure and promotion—and providing structured mentorship and support—ensures sustainability (Mkandawire-Valhmu et al., 2010; Akintade et al., 2025). Embedding anti-racism into faculty development is therefore not just about enhancing teaching, but institutionalising equity and empowering faculty to drive systemic transformation.

4. Partnerships and Co-Creation

Anti-racist nursing and midwifery education must be firmly connected to the wider healthcare and social context. Sustainability depends on genuine partnerships with stakeholders, ensuring curricula remain relevant, grounded in lived experience and responsive to real-world inequities—avoiding siloed, performative or short-term reforms.

Key partners include:

a ***Higher education, healthcare providers and communities:*** Universities, hospitals and clinics must collaborate with local groups to align education with clinical realities and lived experience. Such partnerships provide insight into social determinants of health and effective practice models. Case studies show how embedding community engagement and decolonised curricula strengthens anti-racist education (Betancourt et al., 2003; Council of Deans of Health, 2023).

b ***Educators and regulators:*** Faculty, the NMC and bodies like the Royal College of Nursing (RCN) play pivotal roles in embedding anti-racist pedagogy and assessment, directly shaping inclusive learning.

c ***Students:*** Far from passive recipients, students are essential partners in anti-racist reform. Their feedback exposes how racism manifests in education, while involvement in governance and curriculum design ensures structural competency and praxis. Integrating authentic case studies (e.g., maternal mortality disparities) and Community Based Participatory Research (CBPR) models enable students to interrogate inequities and co-create solutions (Davis et al., 2024; Fleming et al., 2023).

d ***Professional associations and policymakers:*** Government departments, accreditation bodies and professional organisations set equity standards, fund reforms and drive systemic change.

Finally, co-creation through shared governance among students, faculty, communities and professional bodies fosters accountability, mutual respect and relevance, ensuring anti-racist education avoids symbolic gestures (Jeffreys, 2015; Davis et al., 2024).

5. Outcomes-Oriented Evaluation and Continuous Improvement

Effective anti-racist nursing and midwifery education requires robust, ongoing evaluation that measures both process and impact, moving beyond "diversity head-counts" to demonstrate how practice, culture and patient outcomes are transformed (Williams et al., 2019; Benner et al., 2010).

a ***Student outcomes:*** Competency-based assessment should evaluate technical skills alongside critical reflection, advocacy and structural awareness, with patient feedback from clinical sites used to link learning to real-world care (Playfair et al., 2023; AACN, 2009).

b ***Faculty engagement:*** Monitoring professional development, curriculum reform and mentorship ensures anti-racist pedagogy is embedded institutionally rather than dependent on individuals.

c ***Institutional metrics:*** Tracking admissions, retention, progression and leadership diversity—disaggregated by race—exposes equity gaps. In the UK, measures like the awarding gap and NSS scores serve as powerful levers (Iheduru-Anderson & Waite, 2022). Evaluation must also review inclusivity of learning environments and responses to racism reports.

Evaluation should be participatory, iterative and adaptive, engaging students, faculty and communities in shaping frameworks for accountability and relevance. Findings must inform strategy, resources and redesign. Both qualitative (storytelling, case studies) and quantitative measures are vital to capture lived experience and ensure multiple perspectives (Tuhiwai-Smith, 1999; Adichie, 2008). Above all, anti-racism must be recognised as a continuous journey requiring recalibration in response to evolving contexts (Playfair et al., 2023).

Taken together, sustaining anti-racist nursing and midwifery education means embedding equity into everyday teaching, governance and institutional strategy. The Equity Accomplice model transforms commitment into action: educators and institutions actively dismantle racism by taking risks, changing policies and restructuring practices. Training grounded in this model prepares nurses and midwives to deliver equitable, culturally responsive, patient-centred care. Institutional partnerships and resistance strategies reinforce this transformation—ultimately cultivating a workforce that is both clinically excellent and socially just.

Conclusion

Ultimately, it is worth recognising that anti-racism in nursing education is not a destination but a journey. Even so, a journey that is neither quick nor easy but necessary. We believe that whilst individual nursing education contexts may differ globally, the strategies outlined in this chapter provides a good foundation for meaningful action in tackling racism in nursing by addressing how present and future nurses are trained. The strategies outlined in this chapter are by no means exhaustive and we are under no illusion that sustainably implementing anti-racism in nursing education will not be bedevilled with resistance. We are convinced nonetheless that the profession's commitment to its core values is not lost but needs the right steering through the turbulent waters of entrenched systemic racism. As the profession evolves through this journey of anti-racism, research must continue to explore innovative pedagogies that inform practice. Further, the impact of anti-racist education needs to be constantly measured and evaluated in relation to patient outcomes. Finally, individual nurse educators and nursing education systems must hold themselves accountable for progress in ensuring an anti-racism is systemically embedded. The future of nursing and the health of our communities depends on it.

Reflective Activity

Having read the chapter, we invite you to reflect on your key learning and its implications for your professional practice as a nurse or midwife using Bain et al.'s (2002) 5R framework (pp. 13–15):

- Reporting – What is it in your situation you want to transform after reading this chapter?
- Responding – What are your personal observations regarding your own situation/context in relation to what is raised in this chapter?
- Relating – What is/are the theoretical/research/data/legislative, etc., understandings relationship to under consideration in this chapter that you could apply to your situation/context?

- Reasoning – Identify how the chapter findings matter to your situation/context and how will you interrogate your situation/context and what will help you from this chapter?
- Reconstructing – Identify your action plans to reframe and rebuild a transformative way forward to change from the situation in your context.

References

Abayasekara, S.A. (2021). Universal assessment: Reflections on equitable evaluations in a Sri Lankan higher education classroom. *University of Colombo Review (New Series Lll), 2*(1): 102–118. https://ucr.sljol.info/articles/41/files/submission/proof/41-1-76-1-10-20210808.pdf

Ackerman-Barger, K., Boatright, D., Gonzalez-Colaso, R., Orozco, R. and Latimore, D. (2020). Seeking inclusion excellence: Understanding racial microaggressions as experienced by underrepresented medical and nursing students. *Academic Medicine, 95*(5): 758–763. https://journals.lww.com/academicmedicine/fulltext/2020/05000/Seeking_Inclusion_Excellence__Understanding_Racial.30.aspx.

Adichie, C.M. (2008). *The danger of a single story*. TED Talks. https://www.youtube.com/watch?v=D9Ihs241zeg

Akintade, B., Brockett-Walker, C., González, J., Idzik, S., Iheduru-Anderson, K., Indenbaum-Bates, K., Jones, M., Lowery, Y., McCamey, D., Reis, P. & DeWitty, V. (2025). Influence of underrepresented leaders on recruiting and retaining underrepresented faculty and students in nursing programs. *Journal of Professional Nursing, 60*: 123–132. https://doi.org/10.1016/j.profnurs.2025.07.006

American Association of Colleges of Nursing (AACN). (2009). *American Association of Colleges of Nursing-AACN*. https://pesquisa.bvsalud.org/portal/resource/pt/lis-23407

American Association of Colleges of Nursing (AACN). (2021a). *Diversity, equity, and inclusion in academic nursing: Position statement*. https://www.aacnnursing.org/news-data/position-statements-white-papers/diversity-equity-and-inclusion-in-academic-nursing

American Association of Colleges of Nursing (AACN). (2021b). *The essentials: Core competencies for professional nursing education*. https://www.aacnnursing.org/Portals/0/PDFs/Publications/Essentials-2021.pdf

American Nurse Journal. (2024). *Anti-racism in nursing*. https://www.myamericannurse.com/anti-racism-in-nursing

American Nurses Association (ANA). (2022). *National Commission to address racism in nursing: Defining racism*. https://www.nursingworld.org/globalassets/practiceandpolicy/workforce/commission-to-address-racism/final-defining-racism.pdf

Anderson, K.M., Davis, D. and McLaughlin, M.K. (2019). Implementing universal design instruction in doctor of nursing practice education. *Nurse Educator, 44*(5): 245–249. https://doi.org/10.1097/nne.0000000000000642

Bain, J.D., Ballantyne, R., Mills, C. and Lester, N.C. (2002). *Reflecting on practice: Students teachers' perspectives*. Post Pressed.

Bell, B. (2021). White dominance in nursing education: A target for anti-racist efforts. *Nursing Inquiry, 28*(1): e12379. https://doi.org/10.1111/nin.12379

Bell, B.V. (2024). We'd really love to but we're really busy: Silence, precarity and resistance as structural barriers to anti-racism in nursing education. *Journal of Advanced Nursing, 80*(1): 214–225. https://doi.org/10.1111/jan.15795

Benner, P., Sutphen, M., Leonard, V. and Day, L. (2010). *Educating nurses: A call for radical transformation*. John Wiley & Sons. https://books.google.com/books?hl=en&lr=&id=mnI5DwAAQBAJ

Betancourt, J.R., Green, A.R., Carrillo, J.E. and Owusu Ananeh-Firempong, I.I. (2003). Defining cultural competence: A practical framework for addressing racial/ethnic disparities in health and health care. *Public Health Reports*, *118*(4): 293–302. https://journals.sagepub.com/doi/full/10.1093/phr/118.4.293

Bheenuck, S., Miers, M., Pollard, K. and Young, P. (2007). Race equality education: Implications of an audit of student learning. *Nurse Education Today*, *27*(5): 396–405. https://doi.org/10.1016/j.nedt.2006.06.003

Blanchet Garneau, A., Lavoie, P., Sit, V. and Laurent Sédillot, C. (2023). Core components of an anti-racist approach among health professions educators: An integrative review. *International Journal of Medical Education*, *14*: 131–136. https://doi.org/10.5116/ijme.64e9.b6b4

Boakye, P.N., Prendergast, N. and Bailey, A. (2024). Challenging anti-racism in nursing education: A moral and professional call to action. *Nurse Education Today*, *141*: 106305. https://doi.org/10.1016/j.nedt.2024.106305

Boatright, D. H., Samuels, E. A., Cramer, L., Cross, J., Desai, M., Latimore, D., & Gross, C. P. (2018). Association Between the Liaison Committee on Medical Education's Diversity Standards and Changes in Percentage of Medical Student Sex, Race, and Ethnicity. *JAMA*, *320*(21), 2267–2269. https://doi.org/10.1001/jama.2018.13705

Bray, B. (2019). Maslow's hierarchy of needs and Blackfoot (Siksika) Nation beliefs. *Rethinking Learning. https://www.resilience.org/stories/2021-06-18/the-blackfoot-wisdom-that-inspired-maslows-hierarchy/*

Burnett, A., Moorley, C., Grant, J., Kahin, M., Sagoo, R., Rivers, E., Deravin, L. and Darbyshire, P., (2020). Dismantling racism in education: In 2020, the year of the nurse & midwife, it's time. *Nurse Education Today*, *93*: 104532. https://doi.org/10.1016/j.nedt.2020.104532

Caffrey, A., Botticello, J., Quarshie, P.E., Ali, L., Watts, P., Cathala, X. and Ferrante, J. (2023). Student nurses' experiences of discrimination and racism on work placements: What can higher education institutions do? *Nurse Education Today*, https://doi.org/10.1016/j.nedt.2023.105980

Canadian Association of Schools of Nursing (CASN). (2023). *Promoting anti-racism in nursing education in Canada*. https://www.casn.ca/wp-content/uploads/2023/05/Promoting-Anti-Racism-in-Nursing-Education-in-Canada.pdf

Celestini, A. and Palalas, A. (2024). Inclusive online nursing education: Learner perceptions of universal design for learning approaches. *Canadian Journal for the Scholarship of Teaching and Learning*, *15*(3): 2. https://doi.org/10.5206/cjsotlrcacea.2024.3.16911

Coddington, D.M. and Karsten, K. (2014). Eliminating cultural bias in nursing examinations. *Teaching and Learning in Nursing*, *9*(3): 134–138. https://doi.org/10.1016/j.teln.2014.03.002

Council of Deans of Health. (2023). Anti-racism in AHP education: Building an inclusive environment. https://www.councilofdeans.org.uk/wp-content/uploads/2023/03/Anti.racism.in_.ahp_.education.report.pdf

Crenshaw, N., Lewis, L. and Foronda, C.L. (2025). Racism in clinical nursing practice: A qualitative study. *BMC Nursing*, *24*: 105. https://doi.org/10.1186/s12912-024-02521-8

Cressey, J. (2020). Universal design for learning: Culturally responsive UDL in teacher education. In M.T. Grassetti and J. Zoino-Jeannetti (Eds.), *Next generation digital tools and applications for teaching and learning enhancement* (pp. 137–158). IGI Global Scientific Publishing.

Dafny, H.A., Snaith, N., McCloud, C., Waheed, N., Cooper, P. and Champion, S. (2025). Racism during clinical placement, the perpetrators, impact, advocating, and reporting. *Nursing Ethics*, *32*(6): 1886–1899. https://doi.org/10.1177/09697330251317675

Davis, S., Martin-Holland, J., Gemeda, M.L. and Mitchell, D.A. (2024). An anti-racism framework for educating nursing professionals. *Nursing Outlook*, *72*(5): 102242. https://doi.org/10.1016/j.outlook.2024.102242

Day, L. and Beard, K.V. (2019). Meaningful inclusion of diverse voices: The case for culturally responsive teaching in nursing education. *Journal of Professional Nursing*, *35*(4): 277–281. https://doi.org/10.1016/j.profnurs.2019.01.002

Edmonson, A.C. (2018). *The fearless organization*. Harvard Business School.

Fleming, P.J., Stone, L.C., Creary, M.S., Greene-Moton, E., Israel, B.A., Key, K.D., Reyes, A.G., Wallerstein, N. and Schulz, A.J. (2023). Anti-racism and community-based participatory research: Synergies, challenges, and opportunities. *American Journal of Public Health*, *113*(1): 70–78. https://doi.org/10.2105/AJPH.2022.307114

Ford, N.J., Gomes, L.M. and Brown, S.B. (2024). Brave spaces in nursing ethics education: Courage through pedagogy. *Nursing Ethics*, *31*(1): 101–113. https://doi.org/10.1177/09697330231183075

Gonzalez, C.M., Kim, M.Y. and Marantz, P.R. (2021). Implicit bias and its relation to health disparities: A teaching program and survey of medical students. *Medical Education Online*, *26*(1): 64–71. https://doi.org/10.1080/10401334.2013.857341

Hamilton, N., & Haozous, E.A. (2017). Retention of faculty of color in academic nursing. *Nursing Outlook*, *65*(2): 212–221 https://doi.org/10.1016/j.outlook.2016.11.003

Hantke, S., St. Denis, V. and Graham, H. (2022). Racism and anti-racism in nursing education: Confronting the problem of whiteness. *BMC Nursing*, *21*(1): 146. https://doi.org/10.1186/s12912-022-00929-8.

Harris, C. (2018). Reasonable adjustments for everyone: Exploring a paradigm change for nurse educators. *Nurse Education in Practice*, *33*: 178–180. https://doi.org/10.1016/j.nepr.2018.08.009

Iheduru-Anderson, K. and Waite, R. (2024). Decolonizing nursing education: Reflecting on Paulo Freire's pedagogy of the oppressed. *Nursing Outlook*, *72*(4): 102183. https://doi.org/10.1016/j.outlook.2024.102183

Iheduru-Anderson, K. and Waite, R. (2022). Illuminating anti-racist pedagogy in nursing education. *Nursing Inquiry*, *29*(4): e12494. https://doi.org/10.1111/nin.12494

International Council of Nurses (ICN). (2023). *Universal Health Coverage*. https://www.icn.ch/how-we-do-it/campaigns/universal-health-coverage

Jeffreys, M.R. (2015). *Teaching cultural competence in nursing and health care: Inquiry, action, and innovation*. Springer Publishing Company. https://www.researchgate.net/publication/330605220_Teaching_Cultural_Competence_in_Nursing_and_Health_Care_Inquiry_Action_and_Innovation.

Johnson, R., Browning, K. and DeClerk, L. (2021). Strategies to reduce bias and racism in nursing precepted clinical experiences. *The Journal of Nursing Education*, *60*(12): 697–702. https://doi.org/10.3928/01484834-20211103-01

Kavitha, L. (2023). Universal design: Promoting equity and accessibility. *Shanlax International Journal of Arts, Science and Humanities*, *11*(S1i2-Nov): 7–10. https://doi.org/10.34293/sijash.v11iS1i2-Nov.7307

Kendi, I.X. (2019). *How to be an anti-racist*. Bodley Head.

Kishimoto, K. (2018). Anti-racist pedagogy: From faculty's self-reflection to organizing within and beyond the classroom. *Race Ethnicity and Education*, *21*(4): 540–554. https://doi.org/10.1080/13613324.2016.1248824

Kotcherlakota, S., Stamler, L.L., Clark, A. and Howell, M.C. (2024). Implementing universal design for learning in nursing education: Faculty perspectives. *Teaching and Learning in Nursing*, *19*(1): e138–e144. https://doi.org/10.1016/j.teln.2023.10.003

Krieger, N. (2014). Discrimination and health inequities. *International Journal of Health Service: Planning, Administration, Evaluations*, *44*(4): 643–710. https://doi.org/10.2190/HS.44.4.b

Levey, J.A. (2018). Universal design for instruction in nursing education: An integrative review. *Nursing Education Perspectives*, *39*(3): 156–161. https://doi.org/10.1097/01.NEP.0000000000000249

McChesney, K.Y. (2015). Teaching diversity: The science you need to know to explain why race is not biological. *Sage Open*, *5*(4). https://doi.org/10.1177/2158244015611712

Mkandawire-Valhmu, L., Kako, P.M. and Stevens, P.E. (2010). Mentoring women faculty of color in nursing academia: Creating an environment that supports scholarly growth and retention. *Nursing Outlook*, *58*(3): 135–141. https://doi.org/10.1016/j.outlook.2010.02.001

Moorley, C. and West, R. (2022). Inclusivity in nurse education. *Evidence-Based Nursing*, *25*(3): 75–76. https://doi.org/10.1136/ebnurs-2022-103570

National Health Service (NHS) England. (2022). *Combatting racial discrimination against minority ethnic nurses, midwives and nursing associates*. https://www.england.nhs.uk/wp-content/uploads/2022/11/B1897-combatting-racial-discrimination-against-minority-ethnic-nurses-midwives-and-nursing-associates-061222.pdf

National League for Nursing (NLN). (2024). *Combatting racism in nursing education*. https://www.nln.org/detail-pages/news/2024/04/15/combatting-racism-in-nursing-education

Nursing and Midwifery Council (NMC). (2024). *Independent culture review*. https://www.nmc.org.uk/globalassets/sitedocuments/independent-reviews/2024/nmc-independent-culture-review-july-2024.pdf

Playfair, C., Hunt, G. and DaCosta, C. (2023). Developing anti-racist undergraduate nursing education: Themes and action. *British Journal of Nursing*, *32*(15): 746–751. https://doi.org/10.12968/bjon.2023.32.15.736

Puzan, E. (2003). The unbearable whiteness of being (in nursing). *Nursing Inquiry*, *10*(3): 193–200. https://doi.org/10.1046/j.1440-1800.2003.00180.x

Scheirer, T.F. (2021). Using universal design principles in a fundamentals course to promote student transition to nursing education. *Nursing Education Perspectives*, *42*(6): E111–E113. https://doi.org/10.1097/01.NEP.0000000000000672

Sokolowich, J.R. (2025). Unintended consequences—Risk for bias in competency-based assessment. *Nurse Education Today*, *144*: 106404. https://doi.org/10.1016/j.nedt.2024.106404

Suárez-Baquero, D.F.M. (2024). Decolonizing nursing knowledge: Challenging Eurocentrism centring Global South voices. *Nursing Outlook*, *72*(4): 102197. https://doi.org/10.1016/j.outlook.2025.102526

Tuhiwai-Smith, L. (1999). *Decolonizing methodologies: Research and indigenous peoples*. Zed Books.

Verma, A. (2022). *Anti-racism in higher education*. Cambridge University Press.

Walker, C.R., Gunasinghe, C., Harwood, H., Ehsan, A., Ahmed, F., Dorrington, S., Onwumere, J., Meriez, P., Stanley, N., Stoll, N., Woodhead, C., Hatch, S.L. and Rhead, R. (2023). Ethnic inequalities during clinical placement: A qualitative study of student nurses' experiences within the London National Health Service. *Journal of Advanced Nursing*, *80*(4): 1497–1510. https://doi.org/10.1111/jan.15891

Williams, D.R., Lawrence, J.A. and Davis, B.A. (2019). Racism and health: Evidence and needed research. *Annual Review of Public Health*, *40*(1): 105–125. https://doi.org/10.1146/annurev-publhealth-040218-043750

5

PRACTICE EDUCATION

Not Just Equality but an Anti-Racism Approach

Naheeda Rehman and Shadrach Dare*

Introduction

Clinical practice education is the heart of nursing and midwifery training. It is the space where classroom knowledge is put into action, where skills are honed and where professional identity begins to manifest. For many students, placements are both exciting and daunting. The first time they put on their uniform, introduce themselves as "student nurse" or "student midwife" and experience the privilege and responsibility of caring for people at their most vulnerable is a defining step in their journey to becoming a nurse or midwife.

Yet, while practice education is meant to be a site of growth and belonging, for students from the Global Majority, a term that acknowledges the demographic reality that people racialised as Black, Asian or Minoritised in Western contexts form the Global Majority, it is too often a site of exclusion, inequity and racialised harm (Campbell-Stephens, 2021). Their journey through clinical placements is not defined solely by the challenges of mastering skills or managing patient care. Additionally of note, it is shaped by subtle and overt reminders that they are seen as different or less valued (Walker et al., 2024).

This chapter is based on a UK perspective, but the content will be relevant to global communities. This chapter discusses that the aspiration to "treat all students equally" is not enough. Practice education must move beyond a passive stance of equality towards a proactive, intentional commitment to anti-racism. This means recognising the existence of institutional racism in placements, disrupting its reproduction and creating environments where every student, regardless of racialisation

*Note: This chapter was conceived and planned by Naheeda Rehman and Shadrach Dare, but primarily written by Naheeda Rehman.

DOI: 10.4324/9781003565369-5

which includes their intersecting identities, can thrive (Walker et al., 2024). To achieve this, educators, practitioners and regulators must confront uncomfortable truths, question long-standing assumptions and reimagine the cultures of learning that underpin nursing and midwifery (Davis et al., 2024).

The Purpose and Promise of Practice Education

Practice education is a core requirement of nursing and midwifery training. The Nursing and Midwifery Council (NMC) mandates that students complete at least 2,300 hours of direct practice over three years. These placements occur in a range of healthcare settings such as hospitals, community clinics, maternity units and specialist services. Student nurses are under the supervision of qualified professionals who serve as role models, guides and assessors (NMC, 2018a). Each nursing programme has a Practice Assessment Document (PAD) that is used by practice supervisors and assessors to evaluate students' progress. These frameworks break down learning outcomes into domains such as professional values, communication, nursing practice, decision making and leadership (NMC, 2023).

Clinical placements serve a multifaceted purpose that extends beyond the acquisition of clinical skills. According to the NMC's Standards for Student Supervision and Assessment, placements are designed to provide students with high-quality learning, support and supervision during their practice experiences, ensuring they are assessed for both theory and practice learning (NMC, 2023). These experiences are integral to developing professional identity, confidence and a sense of belonging within the healthcare workforce (NMC, 2024). Furthermore, placements offer opportunities to integrate theoretical knowledge with practical application, fostering critical reflection and the cultivation of core values such as compassion, advocacy and ethical responsibility (NMC, 2023). Importantly, placements also function as spaces where students internalise the "hidden curriculum" of professional norms and expectations whether inclusive or exclusionary, which can profoundly influence their trajectory through training (Abbaspour et al., 2022).

Placements are thus both pedagogical and professional social spaces. They are where students learn not only "how to do" but "how to be", how to embody the values, norms and professional behaviours expected of a nurse or midwife (Antón-Solanas et al., 2021). But what happens when those norms are defined in ways that privilege whiteness? What happens when some students are systematically denied equal opportunities to learn, to be heard and to belong? For Global Majority students, the promise of practice education is often compromised by a parallel curriculum of racial exclusion, a "hidden curriculum" that teaches them, implicitly or explicitly, that their presence is tolerated but not celebrated (Miller and Nambiar-Greenwood, 2022).

Racism in Placements

Racism in practice education is frequently insidious, cumulative and difficult to name (Crenshaw et al., 2025). Unlike overt discrimination, it often occurs covertly and subtly in everyday interactions, allocation of tasks or institutional processes that align with whiteness and marginalise Global Majority students (Dancis and Coleman, 2022; Pryce-Miller et al., 2023). Microaggressions are brief, commonplace and often unintentional behaviours or comments, between people, that convey derogatory or dismissive messages about someone's racialised identity, are a pervasive form of interpersonal racism in placements (Sue et al., 2007; Caffrey et al., 2023). Examples include being misidentified, underestimated, excluded from key learning opportunities, or having contributions overlooked. While each instance may appear minor, over time, these acts accumulate, creating psychological stress, decreased confidence and disengagement (Miller and Nambiar-Greenwood, 2022). Whilst more often overt forms of direct racism are dealt with swiftly, the covertness/implicitness of racism makes it harder for students to challenge in our health care settings and for universities to identify and address. Therefore, students need to write down the incidents, in what context they occurred and who was around, so that a pattern or trend can be identified to relate to the legal definitions of racism, discrimination or harassment.

Whilst we seek to understand the racialised experiences of student nurses and midwives, intersecting identities often compound these challenges, shaping the overall picture of inequality. Intersecting identities such as racism, gender, disability and sexuality can all compound the challenges faced by student nurses and midwives on placement, in addition to these protected characteristics, the inherent power imbalance between students and clinical staff can have a profound impact. These dynamics are particularly pronounced for Muslim student nurses, whose intersecting racialised and religious identities can amplify their vulnerability. Social and political changes, such as anti-immigrant policies, heightened media scrutiny of Muslim communities or rising nationalist rhetoric, can exacerbate these pressures by creating an environment of suspicion or bias within healthcare settings (Thorleifsson, 2021). Islamophobia, both overt and covert, can manifest as microaggressions from patients or colleagues, e.g., exclusion from learning opportunities, socialising and teamwork, undermining confidence and professional development. This intersection of racialised and religious identity, combined with broader societal tensions, can make Muslim student nurses and midwives particularly susceptible to stress, isolation and unequal treatment during placements, limiting their ability to fully engage in clinical learning and build professional networks (Abu-Khalaf et al., 2023).

Research has captured the lived experiences of Global Majority students, illustrating how microaggressions manifest in everyday practice.

Unequal Allocation of Opportunities

Many students report being assigned less complex or technical tasks during clinical placements. Walker et al. (2024) describe minoritised student nurses being given fewer hands-on opportunities, less trust from mentors and often asked to perform basic care duties rather than more advanced skills.

Role Invisibility and Misrecognition

Some Global Majority students feel that despite having the same uniform or role, they are not seen as professionals. For example, narratives include being addressed less often by patients or staff, or people directing questions to White colleagues instead of them. The "Where are you really from?" study (Morrison et al., 2023) captured medical students reporting feeling ignored in placements and not being offered the same learning opportunities as white peers.

Hostile or Unsupportive Environment/Silence About Racism

Students sometimes experience discrimination from peers or staff, or bias from patients, and fear negative consequences if they raise concerns. Caffrey et al. (2023) show that student nurses may feel unsafe or unsupported when reporting experiences of racism or microaggressions.

Presumed Incompetence/Exclusion from Informal Learning

Students described assumptions about their capacities (e.g., communication skills) based on racialised identity, which undermines confidence. Informal learning opportunities (shadowing, guided practice) are disproportionately given to White students, while others are left observing more often (Walker et al., 2024)

These subtle, everyday acts of racism have profound consequences. They erode confidence, impact performance and assessment outcomes, decrease engagement with learning, and in some cases, contribute to attrition from nursing and midwifery programmes (Miller and Nambiar-Greenwood, 2022; Walker et al., 2024). Furthermore, the psychological burden of navigating microaggressions sometimes referred to as "racial battle fatigue" can have long-term effects on wellbeing and professional identity (Sue et al., 2007; Hallett et al., 2021).

In summary, racism in clinical placements is rarely dramatic or singular. Rather, it is systemic, cumulative, and often invisible, manifesting through unequal learning opportunities, misrecognition, stereotyping and institutional silence. Hearing the voices of students underscores the urgency of recognising microaggressions and implementing anti-racism strategies to create rights-based inclusive, equitable learning environments where all students can belong and thrive.

Why Racism Persists

Racism in practice education is not accidental but systemic. Several interlocking factors make it a recurring and often invisible feature of student placements.

Historically, nursing and midwifery have been shaped by colonial legacies that continue to influence which knowledge, practices and identities are valued or legitimised (Dancis and Coleman, 2022). Within these frameworks, whiteness frequently operates as the unspoken norm. Standards of professionalism, communication and competence often draw from Eurocentric assumptions, meaning that Global Majority students' risk being judged as deficient simply because they do not conform to these cultural expectations (Walker et al., 2024).

This problem is compounded by a lack of representation. The scarcity of Global Majority staff in senior or supervisory positions perpetuates invisibility, reducing opportunities for students to encounter role models who reflect their own identities (Pryce-Miller et al., 2023). At the same time, the power imbalance inherent in placements means students depend heavily on supervisors and assessors for progression, making it risky to speak up against racism when it occurs (Caffrey et al., 2023). Even when students raise concerns, institutional responses often reflect inertia. Universities and placement providers may prioritise protecting organisational reputation over safeguarding students, addressing complaints through bureaucratic procedures that minimise complaints of racism to devalue them (Dafny et al., 2025). A further layer of complexity arises from insufficient training for supervisors, many of whom lack the confidence or tools to identify and challenge racist behaviour. Consequently, this results in silence to avoid tackling or make invisible the racism, diminishing to discredit or devalue the racism raised, or even gaslighting people into doubting the reality of their experiences/concerns, leaving students without meaningful recourse with the intention to disempower them (NMC et al., 2022).

These overlapping dynamics, historical, cultural, institutional and interpersonal all help explain why racism remains entrenched within practice education. However, understanding why racism persists is only part of the picture. To fully grasp its endurance, we must also consider how these forces are actively reproduced in daily practice and policy.

The persistence of racism in practice education cannot be reduced to historical legacies or underrepresentation alone. It is reproduced through the structures, polices, processes/procedures, practices, silences and cultural norms that shape placements on a day-to-day basis, reinforcing the very dynamics already outlined. One such mechanism is the silence within the curriculum and regulatory frameworks. While earlier we identified insufficient supervisor training as a barrier, the problem extends deeper as national standards rarely mention racism explicitly. This conspicuous omission signals to staff and students alike that racism is not central to professional formation, despite evidence to the contrary (Antón-Solanas et al., 2021).

The lack of robust accountability mechanisms underscores the institutional inertia described earlier. Reporting pathways are often slow, opaque or punitive, effectively reinforcing the sense that speaking out is risky and unlikely to lead to meaningful change (Dafny et al., 2025). Instead of protecting students, these systems sustain the very vulnerabilities that make racism so difficult to challenge. Cultural norms within healthcare also sustain reproduction. As described in the previous section, the biomedical model privileges technical skill over relational or equity concerns. Within this framework, racism is minimised as irrelevant to "real" clinical practice, despite its clear impact on outcomes for both student learning and patient care (Miller and Nambiar-Greenwood, 2022).

Finally, deficiencies in data collection and transparency create the conditions for racism to persist unchallenged. Without disaggregated data on progression and attainment, institutions can claim ignorance of inequities and evading accountability (Pryce-Miller et al., 2023). This lack of visibility closes the feedback loop needed to drive meaningful change. The two are not separate; rather, they operate in tandem, historical and structural forces provide the backdrop, while everyday practices and institutional silences reproduce and normalise racism within placements. Tackling racism in practice education therefore requires interventions that disrupt both persistence and reproduction, dismantling the deep-rooted systems that enable inequity to thrive.

Towards Anti-Racism Practice Education

Addressing racism in practice education requires more than aspirational commitments not only to equality but equity too. As outlined in the previous sections, racism persists and is reproduced through systemic, structural and cultural mechanisms within healthcare and higher education (Arday and Mirza, 2018; Byrne et al., 2020). Clinical placements remain a critical site where students encounter unequal treatment, differential access to learning opportunities and experiences of discrimination that shape both professional identity and future career trajectories (Walker et al., 2024). Tackling these inequities demands a proactive, anti-racism approach that restructures placement cultures, reforms assessment practices and reshapes regulatory oversight. Without such an approach, commitments to equality risk remaining symbolic rather than transformative (Ahmed, 2012).

A crucial step is embedding anti-racism within the professional standards and frameworks that govern practice education. Current policies, such as those of the Nursing and Midwifery Council NMC, acknowledge the importance of inclusion but rarely articulate how racism should be recognised, addressed or prevented in practical terms (NMC, 2018a). This silence creates ambiguity, leaving universities and placement providers without clear guidance and enabling local discretion to substitute for systemic accountability. Scholars have long highlighted that vague appeals to fairness or diversity risk obscuring the specific dynamics of racism, allowing inequities to persist unchallenged (Pilkington, 2018). By contrast, embedding anti-racism into standards would reframe equity as a professional responsibility, positioning it as central to safe and ethical practice rather than as an optional add-on.

One practical mechanism for achieving this is through regulatory audits that extend beyond compliance with generic equality requirements. These could include systematic evaluation of whether placement environments demonstrate active anti-racism practice, for example, through staff training, equitable allocation of clinical learning opportunities and the existence of robust reporting and accountability structures (Amin et al., 2018). Evidence from healthcare workforce studies shows that institutions with clearer accountability structures are better able to identify, challenge and reduce racial inequities (West et al., 2015). Without such standards, however, institutions are likely to continue relying on discretionary practices that vary widely in effectiveness and may reproduce harm (Bhopal, 2018).

Finally, embedding anti-racism in regulatory frameworks also has symbolic and cultural significance. It signals to students, staff and service users that racism is not peripheral but central to questions of patient safety, professional ethics and educational quality. This aligns with wider calls in medical and health professions education for a shift from cultural competence models, which often depoliticise race, towards explicitly anti-racist pedagogies that recognise power, privilege and structural inequality (Metzl and Hansen, 2014). In this way, regulatory reform can act as both a driver of systemic change and a catalyst for shifting institutional cultures towards more equitable and accountable practices. [Note – It has not passed the authors by that the NMC recently was found to be institutionally racist, discriminatory and bullying "NMC commissioned Nazir Afzal OBE and Rise Associates to carry out the review after concerns were raised about the organisation's culture, including racism and fear of speaking up. Over 1,000 current and former NMC colleagues, plus more than 200 panel members who sit on fitness to practise hearings, shared their lived experiences as part of the review. The NMC accepts the report's recommendations" (NMC, 2025)].

Diversifying the Placement Workforce

Representation matters but is not enough and training, monitoring, reviewing and accountability measures are needed too. The underrepresentation of Global Majority staff in supervisory and leadership positions perpetuates exclusionary cultures and denies students role models who reflect their identities (Pryce-Miller et al., 2023). Research indicates that students thrive in environments where diversity is visible in senior roles, both because it signals institutional commitment to equity and because it validates their place within the profession (Walker et al., 2024). Recent studies highlight the impact of representation on student experiences. For example, Global Majority students in UK higher education institutions often face challenges related to culture, representation and barriers to success, including a lack of cultural sensitivity and perceptions of a predominantly White academic culture, which can negatively affect their sense of belonging and academic outcomes (Cook, 2024). Similarly, UNESCO's Global Education Monitoring report emphasises that diverse leadership is essential for shaping inclusive learning environments and that leaders must be supported to act as change agents through fair hiring practices and equitable growth opportunities (UNESCO, 2024).

To address these disparities, *placement providers must commit to recruiting, supporting and retaining Global Majority staff.* This requires not only widening access but also dismantling barriers to promotion and leadership. Universities and healthcare organisations should work collaboratively to ensure Global Majority practitioners are equitably represented across supervisory and educational roles, creating environments where diversity is seen as integral rather than exceptional. Enhancing Global Majority representation in leadership roles is critical for creating inclusive and equitable educational environments. By actively recruiting, supporting and retaining Global Majority staff, institutions provide students with role models who reflect their identities, promoting belonging, validation and academic success (Dawkins, 2021). This does not mean Global Majority staff do not need anti-racism training too, as they can align to whiteness themselves due to its status quo's forceful pull, but the training is necessary for all to sustain an environment safe for Global Majority students to do and be to thrive in an educational context.

Robust Anti-Racism Training: To Mandate or Not

While training alone cannot dismantle structural racism, it provides a critical foundation for change. Research indicates that *many supervisors and assessors lack the knowledge or confidence to intervene when racism occurs*, which often leads to minimisation or silence (NMC et al., 2022). Mandating racial equity training addresses this gap by ensuring all staff receive at least a baseline understanding; however, its effectiveness depends on the content, delivery, the readiness of participants to engage with it and have annual objectives to develop themselves and their services to be proactive in anti-racism accountability.

A key limitation of mandatory training is that it may be less effective if staff are not ready for change or perceive it as a compliance exercise hence no annual accountability objectives attached. When participants are resistant or defensive, training risks being superficial, producing minimal reflection or behaviour change. Research suggests that *transformative learning requires psychological safety*, supporting an environment that has a culture of openness, and willingness to critically examine one's own biases and be able to debate and disagree, conditions that cannot be guaranteed simply by making attendance compulsory (Boakye et al., 2024). In some cases, forced participation can even entrench resistance, with staff disengaging or adopting a performative compliance rather than meaningful engagement. For training to move beyond awareness and produce meaningful change, it must prioritise practical skills, critical reflection and accountability. *Effective anti-racism training should include critical consciousness*, a Freirean term meaning to create and act for change in the world you must expose yourself to the conflicting oppressions in systems that dehumanise, to then deepen knowledge and understanding, only then can you collaborate in social movements to make breaks in the hardened foundation that is the status quo (Freire, 2013). Staff must understand how racism operates both structurally and interpersonally, recognising their own positionality and biases (Dancis and Coleman, 2022). *Culturally safe supervision* should equip staff to support students and colleagues in ways that affirm identity and challenge exclusion (Antón-Solanas et al., 2021). Intervention strategies provide concrete tools for recognising and addressing racism in real time is essential to move from passive awareness to active allyship or proactive acting for change.

Mandating training can be valuable if paired with ongoing evaluation, reflective spaces for community learning and integration into continuing professional development (Caffrey et al., 2023). Without reinforcement or engagement, training risks becoming symbolic rather than transformative, offering the appearance of progress without meaningful organisational reframing and change. Racial equity training is a necessary but not sufficient step toward reducing structural racism. Its effectiveness depends on cultivating readiness, providing safe spaces for critical reflection, and *ensuring accountability within the organisational culture*. When thoughtfully designed and sustained, training can help shift norms and behaviours, but it cannot succeed if staff participation is passive or coerced.

Creating Safe and Accessible Reporting Mechanisms

The persistence of racism in clinical placements is frequently reinforced by *inadequate reporting systems, leaving students feeling unsupported and vulnerable*. Students often perceive complaints of discrimination or racism as unlikely to be taken seriously, while institutional processes are described as opaque, bureaucratic and slow (Caffrey et al., 2023; Dafny et al., 2025). This perception is compounded by *fear that speaking out may jeopardise progression*, placement opportunities or relationships with supervisors, effectively silencing students and allowing discriminatory practices to persist unchecked (Pryce-Miller et al., 2023; Walker et al., 2024). Even when complaints are formally lodged, outcomes are often vague or tokenistic, reinforcing the sense that institutions are unwilling or unable to act decisively (Miller and Nambiar-Greenwood, 2022). To address these issues, institutions must implement confidential, trauma-informed reporting mechanisms that prioritise student safety and psychological wellbeing. Trauma-informed approaches recognise that experiences of racism can have profound psychological impacts, including stress, anxiety and diminished confidence, which may affect learning and professional development (Hallett et al., 2021). *Reporting systems should therefore be designed to minimise retraumatisation*, provide emotional support and ensure that students feel heard and validated.

Anonymous reporting is a critical component of safe and accessible mechanisms. Allowing students to report incidents without revealing their identity can reduce fear of retaliation and increase the likelihood that discrimination is documented and addressed (Dancis and Coleman, 2022). Evidence from healthcare education shows that *anonymous reporting can help uncover patterns of systemic bias that might otherwise remain hidden*, providing institutions with actionable insights for policy and practice improvement (Priest and Williams, 2021). However, while anonymity can protect the reporter, institutions must balance it with the need for effective investigation and follow-up, ensuring that cases are addressed thoroughly even when the reporter's identity is unknown (Antón-Solanas et al., 2021).

Equally important is that reports are investigated promptly and thoroughly, with clear communication to students about the process and outcomes. Providing timely feedback demonstrates institutional accountability and mitigates perceptions that complaints are ignored or undervalued (Dafny et al., 2025). Tailored support for students, such as mentoring, counselling or academic adjustments, is crucial in mitigating the negative impact of incidents on both educational experience and wellbeing (Caffrey et al., 2023). Reporting must also be reframed as a mechanism for systemic improvement rather than a burden on the individual student. Institutions should use data from complaints, whether anonymous or named, to identify patterns, address structural issues and inform policies for equity and inclusion (Priest and Williams, 2021). Anonymised publication of outcomes and trends can enhance transparency, build trust and signal that racism is taken seriously and addressed systemically (Dancis and Coleman, 2022).

Finally, *embedding multi-level accountability into reporting mechanisms ensures that complaints are not only acknowledged but acted upon consistently*. This includes institutional oversight, adherence to NMC standards, and integration with training for supervisors and assessors to reduce the risk of retaliation or informal suppression of concerns (NMC, 2018b; NMC, 2022; Antón-Solanas et al., 2021). Ultimately, effective reporting mechanisms, including confidential and anonymous options, are foundational to creating safe, inclusive and anti-racist clinical learning environments. When students trust that complaints will be taken seriously, addressed transparently can lead to systemic improvement, the culture of silence that perpetuates racism can begin to shift, enabling both individual and organisational growth.

Anti-Racism Assessment Practices

Racism and discriminatory bias embedded in assessment practices reflect how whiteness operates as the norm in evaluating student competence. As noted earlier, power imbalances already make students vulnerable, but *accultural subjective judgements about communication, teamwork or "professionalism" can further disadvantage Global Majority students* when their practices are Eurocentric (Walker et al., 2024). This is particularly evident in the assessment of professional values. While the NMC's Standards of Proficiency (2018) outline core values such as compassion, respect and integrity as essential to safe and effective practice, the interpretation of these values can be highly subjective. Behaviours considered "respectful" or "professional" are often filtered through a Eurocentric lens, which risks disadvantaging Global Majority students whose cultural expressions of respect, authority or collaboration may differ from dominant norms.

The NMC's Standards for Education and Training (2018) make clear that assessments must be fair, evidence-based and inclusive. Standard 1 requires that equality, diversity and inclusion underpin all aspects of learning and assessment, while Standard 3 emphasises the importance of constructive feedback to support student development. In practice, this means that assessment of professional values should avoid relying on tacit and stereotypical cultural expectations and instead be grounded in explicit, transparent criteria that reflect the NMC's universal standards, not localised norms.

The National Education Union (2024), Wales, have a set of principles for anti-racism assessments which is applied here to practice education:

- *Embedding anti-racism formative feedback:* In relation to practice education, it's having clinical supervisors that care to nurture, without racism or bias, their Global Majority students. Feedback "is constructive and supportive, helping students to grow and develop their skills". Supervisors that see their students' embodied culture as a positive enhance their clinical training experience. As opposed to supervisors who try to break the students down to conform to whiteness as the norm.
- *Collaboration and creativity for anti-racism:* When the placement environment is culturally and psychologically safe the students and clinical supervisor will get the best out of their relationship. The interactive experiences between student, clinical supervisor, patient and organisation enable the students and supervisors to bring forward diversity of thought, creativity and innovations in the assessment content.
- *Recognition of diverse narratives*: The assessing clinical supervisor should be culturally humble to work with a diversity of Global Majority students. This will enable the students to include cultural perspectives in their work reflections to enhance their practice and enable professional visibility, belonging and creativity. The different Global Majority students' narratives will assist the professions in understanding and including the varieties in thinking that will provide multiple perspectives to enhance the professions' knowledge, understanding and inform and improve practice and hence, patients' experiences.
- *Addressing intersectionality:* "Assessments should consider the impact of intersectionality, recognising how multiple forms of disadvantage and discrimination can compound and affect students' learning [and assessment] experiences". Paying attention to the systemic "ills" to be able to interrupt/disrupt them to improve the students' practice education experiences and opportunities.

Involving Global Majority students as partners in shaping assessment processes not only increases fairness and fidelity to the NMC standards but also empowers them as agents of change within nursing and midwifery education.

Conclusion: Reflections and Future Directions

Racism in practice education is a pervasive and deeply entrenched issue that cannot be ignored and weakens the nursing and midwifery professions as a whole. Evidence from research and lived student experiences consistently demonstrates that Global Majority students face structural and interpersonal barriers that undermine their confidence, wellbeing and professional development (Caffrey et al., 2023; Pryce-Miller et al., 2023; Walker et al., 2024). Students who experience exclusion, bias or discrimination often face cumulative disadvantages, including poorer assessment outcomes, heightened stress and even attrition from their programmes (Caffrey et al., 2023; Pryce-Miller et al., 2023). We know that these experiences are not isolated incidents more so that they are symptomatic of broader systemic inequities and that they erode the very values at the heart of nursing and midwifery: compassion, equity and person-centred care (NMC, 2018a).

Moving from a model of equality, that is treating all students the same, to a genuine anti-racism approach requires *committed urgent proaction*, a clear recognition of the need and responsibility for action alongside structural transformation at multiple levels of the educational and clinical system (Priest and Williams, 2021; Dancis and Coleman, 2022). Recognising urgent need and *responsibility for action* is essential for leaders, educators and practitioners to confront entrenched *harmful norms*, *take accountability* and ensure meaningful, *impactful and sustainable change*. Structural change is critical to dismantle institutional processes and cultural practices that continue to privilege whiteness and marginalise Global Majority students (Walker et al., 2024). Anti-racism in practice education must be framed as integral to health equity and patient outcomes. By committing to anti-racism as a guiding principle, institutions can ensure that the journey through education is one of empowerment, inclusion and excellence, rather than a survival test against systemic bias. In this way, the professions can uphold their ethical mandate while fostering a diverse workforce equipped to deliver equitable, compassionate care for all patients. Moving beyond mere equality requires recognising the responsibility to address inequities, proactively reform systems and create environments where Global Majority students can thrive without fear of marginalisation. Addressing racism in clinical placements is not only a moral and professional imperative but also a critical factor in advancing public health.

Finally, future directions must focus on transforming placements from sites of survival into environments of belonging, growth and excellence. This transformation requires embedding culturally safe learning environments, equitable mentorship, where feedback and assessment practices are free from bias, transparent and trauma-informed reporting mechanisms, anti-racism curricula and rigorous accountability frameworks (Antón-Solanas et al., 2021; Miller and Nambiar-Greenwood, 2022; NMC et al., 2022). Embedding anti-racism pedagogy into both curriculum and practice, alongside rigorous monitoring and accountability frameworks, can ensure that interventions are meaningful rather than symbolic (NMC et al., 2022). Institutions must also actively co-produce reforms with students, recognising the expertise that Global Majority students bring from their lived experiences. Including student voices in policy development, curriculum design and assessment reform ensures that anti-racism strategies are responsive, practical and effective (Pryce-Miller et al., 2023; Walker et al., 2024). Ultimately, creating placements where all students can flourish is not only a moral and professional imperative rather more essential for the sustainability, credibility and integrity of the nursing and midwifery professions.

Reflective Activity

You are invited to reflect on the chapter and relate to your context using Bain et al.'s (2002) 5R framework.

- **Reporting** – After reading this chapter, what aspects of your current placement, workplace or teaching practice do you feel require transformation? Identify specific instances of inequity, silence or racialised exclusion that you now recognise as requiring change.
- **Responding** – What personal observations do you have when you consider your own experience? Reflect on how the issues raised in this chapter resonate with, or differ from your reality. Consider emotional responses, moments of discomfort or insights that surfaced while engaging with the text.
- **Relating** – Which theories, research findings, policy frameworks or professional standards outlined in this chapter connect most strongly with your situation? How might these perspectives help you interpret and address challenges in your own context?
- **Reasoning** – Why do the issues highlighted in this chapter matter to your situation? Explore how systemic racism or inequity impacts professional development, student learning or patient care in your context. How will you interrogate the practices, structures or assumptions that sustain inequity? Which insights from this chapter will support you in that interrogation?
- **Reconstructing** – What concrete actions can you take to transform your context? Identify strategies to reframe practice, such as advocating for anti-racism policies, challenging inequitable assessment or strengthening reporting mechanisms. Outline an action plan that reflects your role, resources and capacity for influence.

References

Abbaspour, H., Moonaghi, H.K., Kareshki, H. and Esmaeili, H. (2022). Positive consequences of the hidden curriculum in undergraduate nursing education: An integrative review. *Iranian Journal of Nursing and Midwifery Research, 27*(3): 169–180. https://doi.org/10.4103/ijnmr.ijnmr_325_21

Abu Khalaf, N., Woolweaver, A.B., Reynoso Marmolejos, R., Little, G.A., Burnett, K. and Espelage, D.L. (2023). The impact of Islamophobia on Muslim students: A systematic review of the literature. *School Psychology Review, 52*(2): 206–223. https://doi.org/10.1080/2372966X.2022.2075710

Ahmed, S. (2012). *On being included: Racism and diversity in institutional life*. Duke University Press.

Amin, M., Till, A. and McKimm, J. (2018). Inclusive and person-centred leadership: Creating a culture that involves everyone. *British Journal of Hospital Medicine*, *79*(7): 402–407. https://doi.org/10.12968/hmed.2018.79.7.402

Antón-Solanas, I., Tambo-Lizalde, E., Hamam-Alcober, N., Vanceulebroeck, V., Dehaes, S., Kalkan, I. and Huércanos-Esparza, I. (2021). Nursing students' experience of learning cultural competence. *PLoS One*, *16*(12): e0259802. https://doi.org/10.1371/journal.pone.0259802

Arday, J. and Mirza, H.S. (eds.) (2018). *Dismantling race in higher education: Racism, whiteness and decolonising the academy*. Palgrave Macmillan.

Bain, J.D., Ballantyne, R., Mills, C. and Lester, N.C. (2002). *Reflecting on practice: Students teachers' perspectives*. Post Pressed.

Bhopal, K. (2018). *White privilege: The myth of a post-racial society*. Policy Press.

Boakye, P.N., Prendergast, N. and Bailey, A. (2024). Challenging anti-racism in nursing education: A moral and professional call to action. *Nurse education today*, *141*: 106305. https://doi.org/10.1016/j.nedt.2024.106305

Byrne, B., Alexander, C., Khan, O., Nazroo, J. and Shankley, W. (2020). *Ethnicity, race and inequality in the UK: State of the nation*. Policy Press.

Caffrey, A., Botticello, J., Quarshie, P.E., Ali, L., Watts, P., Cathala, X. and Ferrante, J. (2023). Student nurses' experiences of discrimination and racism on work placements: What can higher education institutions do? *Nurse Education Today*, *131*: 105980. https://doi.org/10.1016/j.nedt.2023.105980

Campbell-Stephens, R.M. (2021). *Educational leadership and the Global Majority: Decolonising narratives*. Palgrave MacMillan.

Cook, F. (2024). Representation and sense of belonging for people of the global majority in higher education. *Student Engagement in Higher Education Journal*, *5*(2): 111–128. https://sehej.raise-network.com/raise/article/view/1210

Crenshaw, N., Lewis, L. and Foronda, C.L. (2025). Racism in clinical nursing practice: A qualitative study. *BMC Nursing*, *24*(1): 105. https://doi.org/10.1186/s12912-024-02521-8

Dafny, H.A., Snaith, N., McCloud, C., Waheed, N., Cooper, P. and Champion, S. (2025). Racism during clinical placement, the perpetrators, impact, advocating and reporting. *Nursing Ethics*, *32*(6): 1886–1899. https://doi.org/10.1177/09697330251317675

Dancis, J. and Coleman, B.R. (2022). Transformative dissonant encounters: Opportunities for cultivating anti-racism in White nursing students. *Nursing Inquiry*, *29*(1): e12447. https://doi.org/10.1111/nin.12447

Davis, S., Martin-Holland, J., Gemeda, M.L. and Mitchell, D.A. (2024). An anti-racism framework for educating nursing professionals. *Nursing Outlook*, *72*(5): 102242. https://doi.org/10.1016/j.outlook.2024.102242

Dawkins, D. (2021). Recruitment and retention of minority high school students to increase diversity in the nursing profession. *Nursing Clinics of North America*, *56*(3): 427–439. https://doi.org/10.1016/j.cnur.2021.04.007

Freire, P. (2013). *Education for critical consciousness*. Bloomsbury Academic.

Hallett, N., Wagstaff, C. and Barlow, T. (2021). Nursing students' experiences of violence and aggression: A mixed-methods study. *Nurse Education Today*, *105*: 105024. https://doi.org/10.1016/j.nedt.2021.105024

Metzl, J.M. and Hansen, H. (2014). Structural competency: Theorizing a new medical engagement with stigma and inequality. *Social Science & Medicine*, *103*: 126–133. https://doi.org/10.1016/j.socscimed.2013.06.032

Miller, E. and Nambiar-Greenwood, G. (2022). Exploring the lived experience of student nurses perspective of racism within education and clinical practice: Utilising the flipped classroom. *Nurse Education Today*, *119*: 105581. https://doi.org/10.1016/j.nedt.2022.105581

Morrison, N., Zaman, T., Webster, G., Sorinola, O. and Blackburn, C. (2023). Where are you really from?: A qualitative study of racial microaggressions and the impact on medical students in the UK. *BMJ Open, 13*(5): e069009. https://doi.org/10.1136/bmjopen-2022-069009

National Education Union. (2024). *Anti-racism charter*. https://neu.org.uk/latest/library/anti-racism-charter

Nursing & Midwifery Council (NMC). (2018a). *The code: Professional standards of practice and behaviour for nurses, midwives and nursing associates*. http://www.nmc.org.uk/globalassets/sitedocuments/nmc-publications/revised-new-nmc-code.pdf

Nursing & Midwifery Council (2018b). *Future nurse: Standards of proficiency for registered nurses*. NMC.

Nursing & Midwifery Council. (2023). *Standards for student supervision and assessment*. https://www.nmc.org.uk/standards-for-education-and-training/standards-for-student-supervision-and-assessment/

Nursing & Midwifery Council. (2024). *Independent report finds varied learning experiences for nursing and midwifery students*. https://www.nmc.org.uk/news/news-and-updates/independent-report-finds-varied-learning-experiences-for-nursing-and-midwifery-students/

Nursing & Midwifery Council. (2025). *Independent culture review: Reflection, accountability and action* https://www.nmc.org.uk/about-us/nmc-culture/shaping-our-culture/independent-reviews/

Nursing & Midwifery Council, NHS Confederation & NHS England. (2022). *Combatting racial discrimination against minority ethnic nurses, midwives and nursing associates*. https://www.england.nhs.uk/wp-content/uploads/2022/11/B1897-combatting-racial-discrimination-against-minority-ethnic-nurses-midwives-and-nursing-associates-061222.pdf

Pilkington, A. (2018). *The rise and fall of race equality in higher education*. Palgrave Macmillan.

Priest, N. and Williams, D.R. (2021). Structural racism: A call to action for health and health disparities research. *Ethnicity and Disease*, *31*(Suppl. 1): 285–288. https://www.jstor.org/stable/48667968

Pryce-Miller, M., Bliss, E., Airey, A., Garvey, A. and Pennington, C.R. (2023). The lived experiences of racial bias for Black, Asian and minority ethnic students in practice: A hermeneutic phenomenological study. *Nurse Education in Practice*, *66*: 103532. https://doi.org/10.1016/j.nepr.2022.103532

Sue, D.W., Capodilupo, C.M., Torino, G.C., Bucceri, J.M., Holder, A., Nadal, K.L. and Esquilin, M. (2007). Racial microaggressions in everyday life: Implications for clinical practice. *American Psychologist*, *62*(4): 271–286. https://doi.org/10.1037/0003-066X.62.4.271

Thorleifsson, C. (2021). In pursuit of purity: Populist nationalism and the racialization of difference. *Identities*, *28*(2): 186–202. https://doi.org/10.1080/1070289X.2019.1635767

UNESCO. (2024). *Global education monitoring report 2024/5: Leadership in education—Lead for learning*. UNESCO. https://unesdoc.unesco.org/ark:/48223/pf0000391406

Walker, C.R., Gunasinghe, C. and Harwood, H. (2024). Ethnic inequalities during clinical placement: A qualitative study of student nurses' experiences within the London National Health Service. *Journal of Advanced Nursing*, *80*(4): 1497–1510. https://doi.org/10.1111/jan.15891

West, M., Dawson, J. and Kaur, M. (2015). *Making the difference: Diversity and inclusion in the NHS*. The King's Fund.

6

A STORY OF OUTCOMES FROM EdD RESEARCH ON 'THE INTERNATIONAL NURSE CULTURE AND COMMUNICATION IN THE NHS'

Culture and Communication on the NHS

Michelle Dillon

Purpose of Chapter

This chapter presents key findings from my EdD thesis that explored the experiences of racism and discrimination among internationally recruited nurses working within the National Health Service (NHS). Answering the critical question of how international nurses perceive racism, While the broader study examined the interplay of culture and communication in shaping the professional and personal lives of international nurses, this chapter specifically focusses the perspectives and lived realities of racial bias, exclusion, and systemic inequities. Drawing on qualitative data from semi-structured interviews, the chapter reveals how racism and discrimination, both overt and covert manifest in clinical environments. Participants shared deeply personal narratives that exposed the emotional toll of microaggressions, cultural misunderstandings, and unequal pay banding. These experiences were often compounded by a lack of culturally responsive support and institutional recognition.

Key themes include:

- Microaggressions and Everyday Racism: Subtle yet persistent behaviours that undermine professional identity and reinforce exclusion.
- Structural Discrimination: Limited access to leadership roles, mentorship, and career progression despite qualifications and experience.
- Cultural Isolation: Pressure to conform to dominant norms, leading to identity strain and emotional fatigue.
- Resilience and Advocacy: International nurses often form informal support networks and advocate for equity, despite systemic challenges.

DOI: 10.4324/9781003565369-6

Ethics Approval

This study aligned itself to the ethical research principles of the University of Bath, ethics was approved by The Social Science Research Ethics Committee (SSREC) reference number: S22 132.

Positionality Statement

As a white woman from England, I recognise that my racial identity differs from the internationally educated nurses who participated in this study. This positional gap may raise concerns about bias or misinterpretation. I approached the research with reflexivity and humility, engaging in journaling and prioritising participant voices through direct quotations. Where data interpretation was complex particularly around emotionally or culturally nuanced accounts, I triangulated findings with literature, consulted culturally competent advisors, and revisited transcripts to ensure accuracy. These steps helped uphold the ethical integrity of the study and honour the experiences shared with me.

Background

By 1948, the UK faced a critical shortage of nurses, with 54,000 vacancies prompting the Ministries of Health and Labour to collaborate with the Colonial Office, the Royal College of Nursing (RCN), and the General Nursing Council to actively recruit Caribbean women (Calenda, 2014). That same year, the arrival of the Empire Windrush at Tilbury Docks marked a pivotal moment, as over 1,000 Caribbean passengers disembarked to support Britain's post-war reconstruction efforts. Many from the Windrush generation would go on to play a foundational role in the newly established NHS, filling essential nursing, auxiliary, and domestic roles (Seaton, 2023). Their presence grew steadily, and by 1965, approximately 5,000 Jamaican women were working in British hospitals. By 1977, overseas recruits made up 12% of all student nurses and midwives in Britain, with 66% of those coming from the Caribbean. Throughout the following two decades, Britain's colonies and former colonies continued to supply a steady stream of inexpensive labour to address NHS staffing shortages, although language barriers were cited as a contributing factor to poor retention rates (Snow and Jones, 2011; Seaton, 2023).

Seventy-five years after its founding, the NHS is once again facing a significant workforce crisis (Palmer et al., 2021). In response, both the NHS and the UK government have committed to ambitious targets: reducing the nursing vacancy rate to 5% by 2028 and increasing the number of NHS nurses by 50,000 by 2025. In their report *Return on Investment of Overseas Nurse Recruitment: Lessons for the NHS*, Palmer et al. (2021) emphasise that achieving these goals will require a multifaceted approach. Key recommendations include improving retention rates, expanding support for domestically trained nurses, and implementing initiatives to encourage former NHS staff to return to practice. Crucially, the report acknowledges that addressing the current shortfall will take time, and therefore, the recruitment of international nurses remains an essential and immediate strategy.

According to Baker (2023), 264,822 NHS staff reported a non-British nationality, accounting for 18.7% of all staff whose nationality is known, an increase from 222,107 (16.5%) in June 2022. These individuals represent over 200 nationalities, with Indian, Filipino, and Nigerian staff being the most common among non-British groups. International nurses now play a vital role in delivering high-quality healthcare across England. Nearly one in five (18.5%) nurses working in NHS hospitals and community services is an overseas national, and this proportion is expected to rise. In recent years, overseas nationals have comprised approximately a quarter of new nurse joiners (Palmer et al., 2021). Notably, these figures vary significantly by region. In the Northeast and Yorkshire, 85% of nurses are British, whereas in London, only 60% are. London also has the highest proportion of EU nurses at 10%, while Asian nurses are most prevalent in the East of England, making up 23% of the nursing workforce there (Baker, 2023).

Umbrella Review Findings

An umbrella review was undertaken to examine previously published research on the experiences of internationally recruited nurses within the NHS. Umbrella reviews have gained significant traction over the past decade, largely due to the exponential growth in published research across disciplines. As the volume of systematic reviews continues to rise, umbrella reviews offer a strategic and efficient means of synthesising high-level evidence. According to Aromataris et al. (2020), this methodology is particularly well-suited for examining broad topics where multiple related systematic reviews already exist. It enables researchers to consolidate findings, identify overarching themes, and avoid unnecessary duplication of effort. An umbrella review is a distinct form of systematic review that follows a rigorous, step-by-step process to identify and evaluate the most relevant existing reviews. It accommodates both quantitative and qualitative approaches, making it versatile across diverse research domains (Balante et al., 2021). The primary aim is to provide a comprehensive summary of current evidence while highlighting gaps, inconsistencies, or areas for future inquiry. Given the abundance of empirical studies available on the topic, the umbrella review methodology was deemed appropriate for this research. It allowed for the extrapolation, critical appraisal, and synthesis of key themes across multiple systematic reviews. To ensure methodological rigour, the process adhered to the guidelines set forth by the Joanna Briggs Institute (JBI), as outlined by Aromataris et al. (2020). Drawing on nearly 300 articles from five systematic reviews spanning the years 1995 to 2021, this synthesis identifies recurring themes, evolving experiences, and enduring challenges faced by the international nursing workforce. By consolidating over three decades of evidence, the review offers a comprehensive understanding of the structural, cultural, and interpersonal factors that shape the professional lives of internationally educated nurses. This body of literature provides a robust foundation for exploring the recurring patterns, challenges, and cultural dynamics that continue to influence the integration, representation, and wellbeing of the NHS's international workforce.

The first review, conducted by Nichols and Campbell (2010), is an integrative analysis of 30 studies published between 1995 and 2007. Their work identified five central themes that reflect the transitional and emotional journey of international nurses: (1) *Motivation for migration*, which often stemmed from economic necessity or professional aspiration; (2) *Adapting to British nursing*, highlighting the challenges of adjusting to new clinical practices and workplace expectations; (3) *Experiencing first-world healthcare*, which brought both opportunity and disorientation; (4) *Feeling devalued and de-skilled*, as many nurses reported a lack of recognition for their prior experience; and (5) *Vectors of racial discrimination*, underscoring the systemic and interpersonal biases encountered in the workplace.

Building on this foundation, Moyce et al. (2016) conducted a systematic review of 43 articles published between 1997 and 2013. Their analysis revealed six dominant themes: (1) *Migration and licensing barriers*, which often delayed or complicated entry into the workforce; (2) *Difficulty in communication*, particularly around language and clinical terminology; (3) *Racism and discrimination*, echoing the findings of Nichols and Campbell; (4) *Skill under-utilisation*, where nurses felt their competencies were overlooked; (5) *Acculturation*, reflecting the psychological and social adaptation to a new cultural environment; and (6) *The role of the family*, which influenced both resilience and vulnerability during the migration process.

The third review, Viken et al. (2018), examined 17 studies and distilled three central themes that speak to the sense of alienation experienced by many international nurses: (1) *Being an outsider at work*, where nurses felt excluded from team dynamics and decision-making. (2) *Cultural dissonance*, highlighting the clash between personal values and institutional norms. (3) *Unfamiliar nursing practice*, which created uncertainty and required significant adjustment.

In a more focused analysis, Bond et al. (2020) reviewed six papers and identified four themes that emphasise both the challenges and coping mechanisms of international nurses: (1) *Cultural integration*, which varied widely depending on institutional support; (2) *Individual challenges*, including emotional stress and professional identity conflict; (3) *Support networks*, which played a crucial role in adaptation and wellbeing; and (4) *Communication issues*, reinforcing the importance of language proficiency and cultural literacy.

Finally, Balante et al. (2021) conducted the most extensive review, synthesising over 200 articles. Their findings generated four overarching themes that encapsulate the broader cultural and professional tensions faced by international nurses (1) *Cultural differences*, which influenced clinical interactions and workplace relationships; (2) *Intercultural communication*, often marked by misunderstanding and misinterpretation; (3) *Differing nursing cultures*, reflecting variations in training, autonomy, and expectations; and (4) *Ethnic identity challenges*, where nurses grappled with visibility, representation, and belonging.

Across the five reviews, several cross-cutting insights consistently emerge, shedding light on the complex realities faced by our international workforce within the NHS. Cultural and professional adaptation remains a central challenge, as nurses must navigate unfamiliar healthcare structures, clinical expectations, and workplace norms. Communication barriers, both linguistic and cultural, frequently impede integration, collaboration, and clinical effectiveness, often leading to misunderstandings and professional isolation. Discrimination and marginalisation are persistent issues, undermining nurses' sense of belonging and impacting their professional identity and confidence. Many International nurses report under-utilisation of their skills and feelings of being de-skilled, reflecting systemic barriers to the recognition of international qualifications and prior experience. Finally, support structures, including peer networks, mentorship, and family connections, play a vital role in mediating the migration experience, offering emotional resilience and practical guidance in the face of ongoing challenges. These recurring themes highlight the need for more inclusive policies and culturally responsive practices within the NHS.

Umbrella Review Findings – Racism and Discrimination

While humans do exhibit physical variation across populations, these differences stem from minor genetic distinctions and evolutionary adaptations (Pountney and Maric, 2021). Early scientific attempts to categorise human diversity often relied on superficial traits, resulting in crude taxonomies that reinforced stereotypes and misconceptions (Rutherford, 2017). These classifications laid the groundwork for systemic racism, which has permeated societies globally (Pountney and Maric, 2021). Today, race is widely understood not as a biological reality, but as a socially and politically constructed concept shaped by historical and cultural narratives (Bhopal, 2018). Given the NHS's dependence on an international workforce, it is essential that this construct and its implications is critically examined and taught across all levels of healthcare. Doing so is vital in addressing racism, reducing inequalities, and fostering a more inclusive and equitable working environment.

Nichols and Campbell (2010), Moyce et al. (2016), Bond et al. (2020), and Balante et al. (2021) all identify racism and/or discrimination as a recurring theme in their findings. Nichols and Campbell (2010) report that many internationally recruited nurses experience racial harassment from both colleagues and patients. Similarly, Moyce et al. (2016) document discrimination originating from patients, visitors, peers, and supervisors, highlighting its pervasive nature across workplace interactions. Bond et al. (2020) describe how international nurses often feel distressed, confused, and humiliated due to both overt and covert forms of discrimination. Balante et al. (2021) echo these concerns, suggesting that cultural differences and distinct ethnic identities contribute to marginalisation, which manifests in varied and complex ways across the international nursing workforce.

Nichols and Campbell (2010) further note that international nurses often perceive their visible or cultural differences such as skin colour, language, accent, or perceived foreignness as social markers that make them vulnerable to racial harassment. This led some nurses to question whether they were being empathically recognised as human beings. Marginalisation and social isolation are also explored by Moyce et al. (2016), who quote one Indian nurse stating, "They didn't think I was human," emphasising the emotional toll of such experiences and the dehumanising effects of systemic discrimination.

All four studies, Nichols and Campbell (2010), Moyce et al. (2016), Bond et al. (2020), and Balante et al. (2021) highlight the lack of job opportunities and career progression for international nurses as a form of discriminatory practice. Nichols and Campbell (2010) reveal that international nurses are frequently employed at the lowest grade banding, equivalent to that of a newly qualified nurse, resulting in a loss of professional status and de-skilling. Moyce et al. (2016) note that many of these nurses arrive in the UK with extensive experience and advanced clinical skills yet are often relegated to basic or unskilled tasks until they complete mandatory training, which delays their full integration into the workforce. Bond et al. (2020) echo these findings, reporting that international nurses frequently experience frustration, injustice, and dissatisfaction as their expertise is overlooked, leading to a profound sense of professional stagnation. Balante et al. (2021) further argue that the failure to recognise prior experience and qualifications in remuneration decisions compounds this discrimination, reinforcing a cycle of marginalisation and undervaluation.

Moyce et al. (2016) report that some internationally recruited nurses have experienced overt discrimination in the form of criticism, harassment, and aggression from employers, which has led to financial instability and job insecurity. These experiences highlight how discrimination functions not only as a social injustice but also as a significant barrier to career progression, sometimes resulting in job loss. Bond et al. (2020) further emphasise that international nurses, particularly those who are Black, often face heightened scrutiny from managers and encounter greater difficulty accessing promotions or enrolling in professional development opportunities. Balante et al. (2021) reinforce these findings, noting that international nurses frequently face restricted career growth, including being denied access to training, excluded from leadership and management roles, and systematically overlooked for advancement. Collectively, these studies reveal a troubling pattern of structural inequity that undermines the professional potential and wellbeing of the international nursing workforce.

There should be no place for racism or discrimination within the workplace; however, the findings of this umbrella review reveal a stark contrast to that ideal. Despite the mandatory implementation of Equality, Diversity, and Inclusivity (EDI) training across Higher Education Institutions and NHS Trusts in the UK, the persistence of discriminatory practices both overt and covert suggests that current interventions are insufficient. The lived experiences of internationally educated nurses, as documented across multiple studies, highlight systemic inequalities that continue to undermine professional integration, wellbeing, and career progression.

These findings stress the urgent need for more robust, evidence-informed strategies that move beyond compliance and foster genuine cultural change within healthcare education and practice.

Findings from My Research

The NHS in the UK has relied on an international nursing workforce since its inception in 1948. Despite their essential contributions, previous research has highlighted persistent issues faced by international nurses, including racism, discrimination, unequal pay, and under-representation within the workplace. My study, conducted between September and December 2022, involved one-to-one interviews with six international nurses, whose demographic with a short synopsis is given below. All participants were given pseudonyms. I used Microsoft Teams as the platform for the interviews, this afforded me an instant recording and transcript of each interview. Employing Braun and Clarke's (2022) Reflexive Thematic Analysis, five overarching themes and 15 subthemes were identified. These included: Migration (motivation, preparation, expectations); Culture and Country (food, humour); Culture and the Workplace (work environment, racism and discrimination, nurse-to-doctor relations, nurse-to-patient relations); Communication (mother tongue to English, mother tongue to mother tongue, accents, idioms, slang); and Differences in Nurse Education and Training. As previously stated, this section will focus on Racism and Discrimination that has been experienced.

The six international nurses demographics and short synopsis is given below.

1. Benjie came to London 12 years ago and he was the first to be interviewed. Initially it was just for the pilot study, but I felt it appropriate to include his rich and lived experience of being an international nurse. Benjie currently works in nursing research.
2. Rae was a friend of Benjie, first meeting in nurse training school in the Philippines. She was currently on maternity leave having had her first baby. When at work, she nursed in a neonatal intensive-care unit.
3. Samson travelled to work in London during the COVID pandemic and was by far the youngest of all participants. He currently works on an adult male surgical ward.
4. Jeeva, like Samson, travelled to work in London during the COVID pandemic. She had nursed for the past ten years in Dubai. With 12 years of nursing experience, she currently works on an adult female surgical ward.
5. Bato, with 15 years of nursing experience, has worked in London for the past four years. He had nursed in Libya for three years but had to leave due to the outbreak of war. He currently works on an adult medical ward.
6. Divina, again like Bato, has 15 years of nursing experience, having worked in Saudi Arabia for the past 11 years. She came to London four years ago. Divina currently works in Accident and Emergency care.

Benjie, Rae, Samson, Bato, Jeeva, and Divina like the 30% of London's NHS workforce born outside the UK are entitled to protection under the race-protected characteristic of the Equality Act (2010). Yet, as Adhikari et al. (2023) argue, the lived realities of many internationally recruited nurses tell a different story. Despite their vital contributions to the NHS, nurses from ethnically diverse backgrounds continue to report experiences of discrimination, bullying, harassment, and limited career progression when compared to their White British counterparts. These findings are echoed across the umbrella review, with Nichols and Campbell (2010), Moyce et al. (2016), Bond et al. (2020), and Balante et al. (2021) all identifying racism and/or discrimination as central themes in their research.

In my own study, Divina spoke candidly and at length about the discrimination she has faced in the workplace. She attributed these experiences to indirect racism subtle, systemic, and often unacknowledged forms of bias that shape her daily interactions and professional opportunities. Her account, presented below, offers a poignant and personal lens through which to understand the broader patterns of exclusion and marginalisation faced by many international nurses in the NHS.

> *I think it's indirect racism, it's not exactly attacking you as a person, it's like, for us Filipino's, we're expected to do more... You are expected to do better than the others... We are known to be very hard-working, so they give you 10 patients without a healthcare assistant, so it makes the job harder.*

According to Ahlberg et al. (2019), one of the key reasons racism remains difficult to confront within healthcare settings is that its very existence directly contradicts the professional standards outlined in The NMC Code (2018). The Code mandates that nurses must treat people as individuals, uphold dignity, and challenge discriminatory behaviour. Therefore, acknowledging racism within the NHS not only exposes systemic failings but also implicates institutions and individuals in breaching core ethical obligations. This tension often leads to silence, denial, or minimisation of discriminatory practices, making it harder for those affected to speak out or seek redress.

Table 6.1 summarises the demographics of research participants.

TABLE 6.1 The six international nurses demographics

Participant Name	*Country of Origin*	*Time Qualified*	*Time in the UK*
1. *Benjie*	Filipino nurse Male	14 years	12 years
2. *Rae*	Filipino nurse Female	14 years	12 years
3. *Samson*	Kenyan nurse Male	5 years	1 year
4. *Jeeva*	Indian nurse Female	12 years	1 year
5. *Bato*	Filipino nurse Male	15 years	4 years
6. *Divina*	Filipino nurse Female	15 years	4 years

Divina's account reinforces this reality. She expressed that it is painfully evident how differently international nurses are treated in the workplace. Her experience reflects a broader pattern of indirect racism subtle, systemic, and often unspoken that manifests in exclusion, unequal opportunities, and a lack of recognition. Despite the protections afforded under the Equality Act (2010) and the ethical standards of the NMC, Divina's testimony highlights how international nurses continue to navigate environments where their contributions are undervalued, and their identities marginalised.

> *So, you must focus on your goal and deliver safe patient care, and that's what matters... You don't focus on the other nationalities talking about how you were rendering your care in comparison to them. That's one thing that will be challenging for overseas nurses, it's not just a job, it's how you will do your job.*

Accountability and investment are needed to address institutional racism as a systemic process, that promotes intervention at individual (all staff including leaders and board members making them accountable and responsible for the change), targeted (where patterns and trends are arising shown from data), and universal (through policies and practices to change behaviours and culture) levels, and this should be obvious in any strategic plan (Dorey, 2014). Institutions, companies, and organisations will only invest in something if they are interested in it, as they only measure and act on things they value (Abbott et al., 2016). Structural barriers are historically steeped in racism preventing certain groups of society progressing (Andrews, 2023), Black and Minoritised groups continue to be marginalised despite claims that we live in a post-racial society (Andrews, 2021) as evidenced to the NHS nurse pay banding.

All six nurses interviewed for this study were employed by their respective NHS Trusts on a Band 5 pay scale, the entry-level grade for newly qualified nurses in the UK. This uniform placement is particularly striking given the diverse levels of experience among the participants. For example, Jeeva arrived in the UK with 15 years of nursing experience, yet she too was assigned to Band 5 upon commencement of her role. This practice reflects a broader pattern of professional devaluation, where internationally educated nurses are routinely positioned at the lowest pay grade regardless of their prior expertise. Such standardisation not only undermines their professional identity but also contributes to feelings of frustration, inequality, and exclusion, issues that were echoed throughout the interviews and are consistent with findings from the wider literature. Church (2023a) postulates that when international trained nurses join the NHS, their past expertise from their home countries are not acknowledged, nurses with extensive experience find themselves starting at the lowest level of a Band 5. Thus, corroborating earlier research findings undertaken by Lipuke and Archibong (2013), where Black African nurses who had migrated to work in the NHS had been placed at the bottom on the nursing hierarchy even though they were often better educated and more experienced than their British counterparts. Coumarassamy (Hunter 2023; Church 2023b), in his dual role as Deputy Chief Operating Officer for Birmingham and

Solihull NHS Trust and Chair of the British Indian Nurses Association (BINA), has publicly condemned the widespread practice of under-banding internationally educated nurses. He describes this approach as *morally wrong*, arguing that it fundamentally devalues the essential contributions these professionals make to the NHS. According to Coumarassamy, most NHS providers routinely place international nurses at the lowest point of Band 5, regardless of their prior experience or qualifications. This lack of recognition not only undermines their professional identity but also has a detrimental impact on their morale and wellbeing. He calls for greater accountability from NHS Trusts, urging systemic reform to ensure fairer treatment and proper acknowledgment of international nurses' expertise and service (Devereux, 2023). This critique aligns with broader concerns raised in recent literature and interviews, where experienced nurses like Jeeva who migrated with 15 years of clinical experience were still placed at entry-level pay grades. The issue of under-banding is not just a bureaucratic oversight; it reflects deeper structural inequities that perpetuate professional marginalisation.

The willingness of nurses like Samson to engage with patients, even in moments of linguistic disconnect, reflects a profound commitment to care and connection. His response to being laughed at, turning the moment into a learning opportunity demonstrates emotional intelligence and adaptability

> *I had this patient who used to speak slang. Cockney English, he used to joke with me a lot and laugh at me because he knew I didn't get anything he said. So I used to tell him, put it in simple English and then maybe at the end of the shift you can teach me your English.*

This reflection captures a deeply nuanced reality one where humility, resilience, and professionalism coexist with subtle forms of exclusion. Yet, it also highlights how indirect racism, often masked as "banter," remains embedded in workplace interactions. Samson's experience is not isolated. The use of regional slang or culturally specific humour, when weaponised or used to highlight difference, can reinforce feelings of otherness. While some may dismiss such moments as harmless jokes, for international nurses they often serve as reminders of their outsider status. The expectation to decode unfamiliar language while maintaining professionalism adds an invisible layer of labour one that is rarely acknowledged.

Recognising this dynamic is crucial, the humility shown by international nurses in navigating these interactions should be celebrated, but the underlying structures that normalise exclusionary "banter" must also be challenged. Creating a workplace culture where linguistic diversity is respected and where humour does not come at the expense of dignity is essential for fostering true inclusivity in the NHS.

In January 2024, Kline and Warmington published their landmark report *Too Hot to Handle? Why Concerns About Racism Are Not Heard or Acted On*, which exposes the persistent and systemic nature of race discrimination within the NHS. Drawing on insights from significant employment tribunal cases and over 1,300 responses from NHS staff, the report paints a sobering picture of the institutional barriers faced by racially minoritised employees.

Key findings from the executive summary include:

- UK-trained staff are significantly more likely than internationally trained staff to raise concerns about racism.
- The most cited reason for not raising a concern was the belief that doing so would not lead to change.
- Of those who did raise concerns, only 5.4% felt they were taken seriously.
- In the majority of cases, no action was taken in response to the complaint.
- Alarmingly, 5.0% of individuals who raised concerns were themselves subjected to disciplinary action.
- 41.8% of respondents reported leaving their jobs due to the treatment they received.

These findings emphasise the urgent need to embed anti-racism education within pre-registration nursing programmes and broader healthcare training. Home students must be equipped not only with clinical competence but also with the cultural awareness and moral courage to advocate for equity and justice within the NHS. The next generation of healthcare professionals must be prepared to support and stand alongside both the UK's Black and Minority ethnic communities and internationally recruited staff groups that remain essential yet underrepresented and undervalued. As the authors of the report aptly note, the NHS, like many institutions, reflects the broader societal discomfort with confronting racism. Despite the proliferation of "toolkits" and policy frameworks, what is sorely lacking is the *practice* of engaging in difficult, honest conversations about race, power, and accountability. Without this cultural shift, efforts to address discrimination will remain superficial, and the lived experiences of minoritised staff will continue to be dismissed or denied.

In July 2024, the Nursing and Midwifery Council (NMC) released the findings of its *Independent Culture Review*, conducted by Rise Associates under the leadership of Nazir Afzal OBE. The review examined workplace culture across the organisation over the previous five years. During a five-month period, 1,044 employees completed an online survey, supplemented by interviews with current staff, NMC panel members, focus groups, and hundreds of confidential submissions via a secure email channel. These included personal accounts, documents, and letters from NHS staff detailing their experiences of discrimination, bullying, and exclusion. As Afzal (2024) stated, "This is one of the most thorough investigations into the culture of a UK health regulator, and the high levels of engagement reflect a sense of emergency among staff to restore a clear sense of purpose and push through reforms that are long overdue." Among the review's key recommendations was the urgent development of an *Anti-Racist Action Plan* to ensure racial equity, rebuild trust between staff groups, and recognise the contributions of Black and Minority ethnic professionals. Crucially, the report emphasised that implementation would require deep and sustained cultural and behavioural change, grounded in the NMC's core values: *Prioritise People, Practise Effectively, Preserve Safety, and Promote Professionalism and Trust.* These themes outline what good practice looks like, emphasising putting patient and service user interests first, providing safe and effective care, and fostering trust through professionalism.

These findings resonate strongly with the experiences of Benjie, Rae, Samson, Bato, Jeeva, and Divina, whose testimonies in this study reflect the same patterns of systemic racism, marginalisation, and institutional neglect. When viewed alongside the evidence presented by Kline and Warmington (2024), a clear picture emerges: racism in healthcare is not an anomaly, it is embedded within structures, policies, and everyday interactions. Despite the NHS's public commitment to equality, the reality for many international and racially minoritised staff is one of exclusion, under-recognition, and harm.

Our collective understanding of race remains constrained by outdated stereotypes tied to ethnicity, religion, and culture. It is essential to acknowledge that race is a socially constructed concept one shaped by power, history, and ideology. Current approaches to diversity and inclusion often fail to interrogate these deeper structures, leaving personal and organisational belief systems unchallenged. If meaningful change is to occur, it must begin with a shift in consciousness, followed by systemic reform across education, regulation, leadership, and accountability.

The findings of this study reinforce a troubling reality: while the NHS remains heavily reliant on its international nursing workforce, these professionals continue to face entrenched systemic challenges. Racial discrimination, pay disparities, and limited representation persist particularly when compared to less experienced, White, UK-born colleagues. Such inequities stand in stark contrast to the foundational principles of nursing, which include equality, respect, and cultural competence. Discrimination in any form constitutes a direct violation of core nursing ethics and its consequences are far-reaching compromising patient care, eroding staff wellbeing, and undermining the integrity of the healthcare system itself.

Change

If the UK continues to recruit internationally educated nurses into its healthcare system, then it must also commit to safeguarding their wellbeing, dignity, and professional equity. The evidence laid out in this chapter makes clear that racism whether overt, covert, or structural is embedded within the NHS and continues to harm those who have come to serve it. Addressing this is not the responsibility of one group alone; it requires coordinated action across multiple levels of the system. Change must begin in pre-registration nurse education, where students are given the space to explore their positionality and engage critically with issues of racism, power, and privilege. But it must also extend to key nursing leaders, including the

Royal College of Nursing (RCN) and the NMC, who must take a more active role in setting anti-racism standards, enforcing accountability to deliver on and measure anti-racism strategic actions, and amplifying the voices of and collaborating with international nurses. Chief executives, board members, and senior managers within NHS Trusts must move beyond performative commitments and embed anti-racist policies into the fabric of their organisations. This includes implementing robust mechanisms to record, investigate, and act on incidents of racism, with clear outcome measures and transparent reporting structures that hold individuals and institutions to account. Only by recognising racism as a systemic issue and responding with systemic solutions can the NHS begin to heal the harm it has caused and build a future where every nurse, regardless of origin and heritage, is valued, protected, and empowered.

Conclusion

Anti-racism change is about a willingness to listen deeply, to be guided by, and to stand in solidarity with those whose voices have historically been marginalised or silenced. Then ACT, this is urgent and necessary for change for the nurses that are experiencing racism. In the context of international nursing within the NHS, this means recognising the lived experiences of racism and discrimination not as isolated incidents, but as systemic patterns that demand critical reflection and structural change. Anti-racism in nursing, and in general any healthcare, education, and practice require us to move beyond tokenistic inclusion and towards genuine co-creation of knowledge and policy. It invites educators, practitioners, and policymakers to interrogate whose perspectives are privileged, whose are excluded, and how power operates within these dynamics to enable and sustain intersectional racism.

Drawing on the findings of this doctoral research, it advocates for change rooted in education, accountability, and cultural humility. By embedding anti-racism pedagogy into pre-registration nurse education, reforming recruitment and progression practices, and fostering anti-racism inclusive workplace cultures, the NHS can begin to dismantle the structures that perpetuate inequality. To recruit is to take responsibility not only for employment, but for wellbeing, dignity, and justice. Anything less is a betrayal of the values the NHS claims to uphold.

Reflective Activity

Having read the chapter, we invite you to reflect on your key learning and its implications for your professional practice as a nurse or midwife using Bain et al.'s (2002) 5R framework (p. 13–15):

- Reporting – What is it in your situation you want to transform after reading this chapter?

- Responding – What are your personal observations regarding your own situation/context in relation to what is raised in this chapter?
- Relating – What is/are the theoretical/research/data/legislative, etc., understandings relationship to under consideration in this chapter that you could apply to your situation/context?
- Reasoning – Identify how the chapter findings matter to your situation/context and how will you interrogate your situation/context and what will help you from this chapter?
- Reconstructing – Identify your action plans to reframe and rebuild a transformative way forward to change from the situation in your context.

References

Abbott, K., Green, J., and Keohane, R. (2016). Organizational ecology and institutional change in global governance. *International Organization, 70*(2), 247–277. https://www.jstor.org/stable/24758325

Adhikari, R., Corcoran, J., Smith, P., Rodgers, S., and Suleiman, R. (2023). It's ok to be different: Supporting Black and minority ethnic nurses and midwives in their professional development in the UK. *Nurse Education in Practice, 66*, 103508. https://doi.org/10.1016/j.nepr.2022.103508

Afzal, N. (2024). *The nursing and midwifery council. Independent Culture Review*. Rise Associates and the NMC UK.

Ahlberg, B., Hamed, S., Thapar-Bjorert, S., and Bradby, H. (2019). Invisibility of racism in the global neoliberal era: Implications for researching racism in healthcare. *Frontiers in Sociology, 4*(61), 1–9. https://doi.org/10.3389/fsoc.2019.00061

Andrews, K. (2021). *The New Age of Empire. How Racism and Colonialism Still Rule the World*. Penguin Books UK.

Andrews, K. (2023). *The Psychosis of Whiteness, Surviving the Insanity of a Racist World*. Allen Lane UK.

Aromataris, E., Fernandez, R., Godfrey, C., Holly, C., Khalil, H., and Tungpunkom, P. (2020). Umbrella reviews. *Manual for Evidence Synthesis. JBI, 2024*. https://doi.org/10.46658/JBIMES-24-08; https://synthesismanual.jbi.global https://synthesismanual.jbi.global

Bain, J.D., Ballantyne, R., Mills, C., and Lester, N.C. (2002). *Reflecting on Practice: Students Teachers' Perspectives*. Post Pressed.

Baker, C. (2023). *NHS staff from overseas: Statistics*. House of Commons, Library Briefing Paper 7783 UK.

Balante, J., van den Broek, D., and White, K. (2021). How does culture influence work experience in a foreign country? An umbrella review of the cultural challenges faced by internationally educated nurses. *International Journal of Nursing Studies, 118*, 103930. https://doi.org/10.1016/j.ijnurstu.2021.103930

Bhopal, K. (2018). *White Privilege, the Myth of Post Racial Society*. Policy Press.

Bond, S., Merriman, C., and Walthall, H. (2020). The experience of international nurses and midwives transitioning to work in the UK: A qualitative synthesis of the literature from 2010 to 2019. *International Journal of Nursing Studies, 110*, 103693. https://doi.org/10.1016/j.ijnurstu.2020.103693

Braun, V. and Clarke, V. (2022). *Thematic Analysis. A Practical Guide*. Sage Publications UK.

Calenda, D. (2014). *Investigating the Working Conditions of Filipino and Indian-Born Nurses in the UK. ILO Asia-Pacific Working Papers Series*. International Labour Organisation Philippines.

Church, E. (2023a). *Health secretary 'aware' of under-banding of overseas nurses*. https://www.nursingtimes.net/news/workforce/health-secretary-aware-of-under-banding-of-overseas-nurses-21-06-2023/

Church, E., (2023b). Overseas nurses facing unexpected challenges: NT. *Nursing times, (magazine)*, *119*(6), 6–7. https://www.proquest.com/docview/3050282001?sourcetype=Magazines

Dorey, P. (2014). *Policy Making in Britain: An Introduction*. Sage Publications UK.

Equality Act. (2010). https://www.legislation.gov.uk/ukpga/2010/15/contents

Hunter, W. (2023). 'BAME people don't have enough voice in the system' says British Indian Nurses Association founder. *Nursing In Practice* 15 March https://www.nursinginpractice.com/latest-news/bame-people-dont-have-enough-voice-in-the-system-says-british-indian-nurses-association-founder/

Kline, R. and Warmington, J. (2024). Too Hot to Handle? Why Concerns About Racism Are Not Heard or Acted on. BRAP. https://27aa994b-a128-4a85-b7e6-634fb830ed15.usrfiles.com/ugd/27aa99_9a9468c5e4da43288da375a17092d685.pdf

Likupe, G. and Archibong, U. (2013). Black African nurses experience of equality, racism, and discrimination in the national health service. *Journal of Psychological Issues in Organisational Culture*, *3*(S1), 227–246. https://doi.org/10.1002/jpoc.21071

Moyce, S., Lash, R. and Siantz, M. (2016). Migration experiences of foreign educated nurses: A systematic review of the literature. *Journal of Transcultural Nursing*, *27*(2), 181–188. https://doi.org/10.1177/1043659615569538

Nichols, K. and Campbell, J. (2010). The experiences of internationally recruited nurses in the UK (1995–2007): An integrative review. *Journal of Clinical Nursing*, *19*, 2814–2823. https://doi.org/10.1111/j.1365-2702.2009.03119.x

Nursing and Midwifery Council (NMC). (2018). *The Code: Professional Standards of Practice and Behaviour for Nurses, Midwives, and Nursing Associates*. NMC.

Palmer, B., Leone, C., and Appleby, J. (2021). *Return on Investment of Overseas Nurse Recruitment: Lessons for the NHS*. Nuffield Trust.

Pountney, L. and Maric, T. (2021). *Introducing Anthropology*. 2nd edition. Polity Press

Rutherford, A. (2017). *A Brief History of Everyone Who Ever Lived*. W&N UK.

Seaton, A. (2023). *Our NHS, a History of Britain's Best Institution*. Yale University Press.

Snow, S. and Jones, E. (2011). Immigration and the National Health Service: Putting history to the forefront. *History and Policy*. https://historyandpolicy.org/policy-papers/papers/immigration-and-the-national-health-service-putting-history-to-the-forefron/

Viken, B., Solum, E., and Lyberg, A. (2018). Foreign educated nurses' work experiences and patient safety: A systematic review of qualitative studies. *Nursing Open*, *5*(4), 455–468. https://doi.org/10.1002/nop2.146

7

THE WELSH POLICY STORY

Anti-Racism and Leadership Challenges in Nursing

Sue Tranka, Richard Desir, and Anton Emmanuel

Introduction

Nursing in Wales, United Kingdom has enjoyed the support and contribution of global majority nurses since its inception (Cummings & Serrant, 2018; Peate, 2024) yet it has not made in-roads to break the glass ceilings entrenched in the structures of the health service, to aid the progression of those nurses into leadership position for the last two decades (Lanada & Culligan, 2024).

Wales is a constituent country of the United Kingdom, home to approximately 3.2 million people. It is distinguished by its rich cultural heritage and bilingual population. The country faces demographic shifts, including an ageing population, which presents both opportunities for public services, healthcare, and community planning. The nation is committed to inclusive governance, sustainable development, and enhancing the wellbeing of its citizens, with a particular focus on rural resilience, digital innovation, and equitable access to services.

Wales has encountered healthcare workforce opportunities that mirror global trends. In response, strategic international recruitment has brought nurses from countries including the Philippines, India, Africa, Europe, and other parts of Asia (Welsh Government, 2023; NHS Wales Shared Services Partnership, 2023). Additionally, individuals from global majority backgrounds, particularly second-generation communities in the UK—are increasingly represented in the healthcare workforce (Dustmann et al., 2010).

The Nursing Workforce in Wales

In 2025, Wales had a workforce of 41,452 nurses and midwives employed in both health and social care sectors. The percentage of professionals from the global majority was 13.7%, an increase from 9.5% in 2020.

DOI: 10.4324/9781003565369-7

According to the most recent census data, 6.2% of the population in Wales identify as belonging to the global majority (Office for National Statistics, 2022).

This indicates that the National Health Service (NHS) workforce—of which Nurses and midwives represent the largest professional group within the NHS workforce in Wales, accounting for approximately 40% of the total (NHS Wales Shared Services Partnership, 2023). Notably, the proportion of staff from global majority backgrounds within the NHS is now more than double their representation of the general population. This pattern reflects similar trends observed in England (NHS England, 2021). However, increased representation does not equate to parity of experience. Most notably, individuals from global majority backgrounds remain significantly underrepresented in middle and senior leadership roles—a disparity that has persisted over several years (NHS Wales WRES, 2024; Kapadia et al., 2022).

The global majority nursing workforce in Wales encompasses both internationally educated nurses (IENs)—those born and trained outside the UK—and UK-educated nurses from global majority backgrounds, often referred to as first- and second-generation professionals. In 2025, approximately 21% of new registrants in Wales were internationally educated, representing a significant portion of the global majority workforce (NMC, 2025). While this figure highlights the impact of international recruitment, it does not fully capture the total proportion of new registrants from global majority backgrounds, which also includes UK-educated individuals. Although the exact percentage is not specified, it is likely higher, reflecting broader demographic shifts and increasing diversity within the nursing profession.

Later-generation immigrants frequently enter the healthcare workforce (Race Disparity Unit, Equality Hub, 2023), partly due to well-established evidence showing that second-generation children in the UK often outperform their white British peers in education—particularly at higher education levels—despite coming from more disadvantaged socioeconomic backgrounds (Dustmann et al., 2010). While this group generally experiences greater upward social mobility compared to their parents, their employment outcomes—especially among university-educated individuals such as nurses—remain lower than those of white British citizens. This suggests that second-generation immigrants, including those with UK-obtained nursing degrees, face significant areas for growth to entering the labour market and work hard to translate their educational achievements into access to high-skilled employment (Di Iasio et al., 2024). These opportunities differ from those faced by IENs but nonetheless contribute to the broader picture of racial inequity reflected in workforce data.

Second Generation Global Majority Nurses and International Educated Nursing Workforce

While the nursing literature in the UK has historically focused on IENs, there is a growing recognition of the need to differentiate and support second-generation global majority nurses—UK-born children of immigrants—who make up a significant proportion of the global majority workforce.

There is currently limited research focused specifically on second-generation global majority nursing staff in the UK. Most literature either groups all global majority nurses together or concentrates on IENs. For instance, reviews by West and Nayar (2016), Mashinkila et al. (2023), and Sanches et al. (2024) did not differentiate between UK-born second-generation staff and IENs. Dustmann et al. (2010) found that second-generation ethnic minorities often outperform their White British peers academically yet continue to face lower employment rates and wage disparities, particularly among men.

In contrast, IENs face opportunities related to cultural adaptation, language areas for growth, and qualification recognition. Much of the nursing literature focuses on pastoral support for IENs, such as integration and onboarding, with developing attention to long-term career progression.

Despite their differences, both groups share common opportunities: underrepresentation in leadership, systemic bias, and developing access to informal networks and sponsorship. Both require tailored policy interventions and leadership development frameworks.

Table 7.1 summarises the key similarities and differences between the two groups:

TABLE 7.1 Comparative analysis: Second-generation global majority staff vs. internationally educated nurses (IENs)

Dimension	*Second-Generation Global Majority Staff*	*Internationally Educated Nurses (IENs)*	*Similarities*
Origin & Education	UK-born, educated in UK schools and universities. Often outperform White British peers in education (Dustmann et al., 2010).	Educated abroad, often with strong clinical skills but different curricula (Dahl et al., 2022).	Both groups are part of the global majority workforce and face systemic barriers despite qualifications.
Early Challenges	Face early educational disadvantages (e.g., language, socioeconomic factors) but catch up and excel by Key Stage 4 (Dustmann et al., 2010).	Face challenges in adapting to UK systems, language, and clinical expectations (Tamburello et al., 2025).	Both require support structures to overcome initial disadvantages.
Employment Outcomes	Despite higher education, experience lower employment rates and wage disparities, especially among men (Dustmann et al., 2010).	Often employed at Band 5 level; face limited progression and wage disparities (Lanada & Culligan, 2024).	Both groups are underrepresented in leadership and face wage gaps compared to White British peers.

(*Continued*)

TABLE 7.1 (Continued)

Career Progression	Lack of visibility in workforce planning; rarely targeted in leadership programmes.	Often receive pastoral support but not career development or leadership training.	Both face barriers to progression and are underrepresented in senior roles.
Policy Attention	Rarely differentiated in workforce data or policy. Often grouped under broad global majority categories.	Well-documented in recruitment strategies; focus on integration, not advancement.	Both need tailored policy interventions and data disaggregation.
Cultural Integration	Culturally fluent in UK norms but still face stereotyping and systemic bias.	Require cultural adaptation and support to navigate UK systems.	Both experience discrimination and exclusion in workplace culture.

Implications for Nursing and Midwifery

- Policy Differentiation: Workforce planning must distinguish between IENs and second-generation staff to address their unique opportunities.
- Leadership Development: Programmes should be inclusive of both groups, with tailored pathways that reflect their backgrounds and needs.
- Data Disaggregation: WRES and other datasets should track generational status to inform targeted interventions.
- Structural Reform: Move beyond pastoral support to systemic change that tackles bias and exclusion.

Enter the Anti-Racist Wales Action Plan (ARWAP)

The Nursing profession is at the forefront of patient care, playing an essential role in shaping health outcomes and addressing systemic inequalities. In Wales, the ARWAP, launched in 2022 (Welsh Government, ArWAP, 2022) represents a landmark commitment to creating a nation free from systemic racism. Central to this mission is transforming healthcare, including nursing to ensure fairness and equity in both workforce practices and patient care. This chapter explores the ARWAPS impact on nursing and midwifery, outlining progress made, opportunities faced, and the path forward to achieving an anti-racism healthcare system where the professions can flourish. It was with a deep sense of responsibility that the Chief Nursing Officer (CNO) published in the first year a set of priorities for the nursing and midwifery placing a focus and need for Professional Equity for nurses and midwives from a global ethnic majority background, whilst equitably improving health outcomes for all, amongst four other priorities (Welsh Government, CNO Priorities, 2022).

ARWAP Objectives

The ARWAP is a comprehensive strategy that recognises systemic racism as a key determinant of health differences to be addressed and workplace inequalities. For nursing the plan outlines specific objectives that emphasise workforce diversity, culturally competent care, and the creation of inclusive environments for both staff and patients. This was a pivotal moment for the nursing profession in Wales, a plan with significant implications, promising and guiding efforts to create a more inclusive and equitable healthcare environment. This strategic plan has aligned seamlessly with renewed leadership in Wales, marked by the appointment of the CNO, Nursing Officers from the global majority, and the implementation of the Workforce Race Equality Standard (WRES). The profession in Wales was thrust into an awakening, contemplating new language and nomenclature, feeling safe to spotlight inequality, and sharing stories of need for progression in global ethnic majority workforce. That all this occurred during the COVID-19 pandemic was a quirk of fate—the pandemic had an unequivocal uneven effect on global majority people, amplifying pre-existing inequality in society and the workforce (NHS Confederation, 2022; NHS England, 2021). This combination of the global pandemic and the direction-setting of the Welsh Government has sharply focused on the ambitions of the country regarding the NHS workforce.

The Impact of the COVID-19 Pandemic

That these senior personnel changes occurred during the COVID-19 pandemic was a quirk of fate—one that added urgency and visibility to the topics for enhancement of inequality and workforce reform. The pandemic had an unequivocal uneven effect on the global majority people (NHS England, 2021) amplifying pre-existing inequality in society and the workforce (NHS Confederation, 2022). This adversely impacted career advancement, employment stability, and the overall workplace experiences of global majority staff (Rhead et al., 2024). Additionally, staff perceived a need for adequate protection and racially inequitable treatment which diminished trust in employers and the broader NHS among some global majority staff (NIHR Evidence, 2022). Global majority staff reported feeling pressured to remain in high-possibility roles despite personal safety concerns (Kapilashrami et al., 2022). Experiences of bias and unfair treatment based on ethnicity further harmed the mental and physical wellbeing of Black and global majority people during the pandemic. Strikingly, global majority healthcare workers were at higher possibility of contracting COVID-19 and experiencing severe outcomes, including death (Rhead et al., 2024). This combination of the global pandemic and the direction-setting of the Welsh Government has sharply focussed the ambitions of the country about the NHS workforce.

Impact of Leadership

The impact of leadership that reflects and represents the diversity of the workforce cannot be overstated. Such leadership brings hope, validates lived experiences of inequality, and affirms the need for change. It creates space for voices that were previously unheard, supports career progression, and advocates for those who have long been marginalised. When leaders are intentional about fostering fairness, equity, and opportunity, they lay the foundation for a culture of growth, inclusion, and innovation.

The Francis Report (2013), following the Mid-Staffordshire scandal, exposed how leadership focused on system performance over patient care fostered a harmful culture. It serves as a cautionary example of what happens when leadership fails to prioritise staff wellbeing and patient dignity, reinforcing the need for inclusive, value-driven leadership that centres people at its core.

The combined efforts from Government policy, national leadership and the first ever Welsh NHS data collection via the WRES data set has illustrated the limited presence of leadership positions in the health service held by global majority staff. The data whilst notable, and revealing is not altogether surprising, nor is this its unique position when compared to WRES data in England (NHS England, WRES, 2024).

Effective Governance, Accountability Structures

Drawing on lessons from NHS England, Welsh WRES governance ensures a robust action and accountability framework.

Welsh Ministers have used their powers to ensure NHS organisations demonstrate tangible anti-racist leadership. Since 2023 Welsh Government have required all NHS Board Chairs to have anti-racist objectives.

All NHS organisations have appointed executive equality champions and formulated local anti-racism action plans.

NHS organisations are required to address WRES data through their Strategic Equality Plan reporting cycle to the Welsh Government. With extensive feedback provided to pinpoint impactful local actions to tackle these essential topics for enhancement. Progress is further scrutinised through the established NHS Planning and Performance mechanisms.

NHS Wales WRES

The launch of the NHS Wales Workforce Race Equality Standard in NHS Wales is a significant milestone in the Welsh Government's Anti-Racist Wales Action Plan (ARWAP), introduced in 2022. The WRES is a key priority in the ARWAP which has been a programme for government commitment for Welsh Ministers since 2022, with the aim of ensuring Wales is an anti-racist nation by 2030. Collecting detailed workforce data to accurately pinpoint actions needed by each organisation as a precursor to ensuring accountability is at the heart of what the WRES for Wales aims to achieve. In its first stage, work has focused on gathering data from each of the NHS Wales's Health Boards, Trusts, and Special Health Authorities on how they are performing on indicators related to race and comparing this nationally. The WRES aims to address racial differences to be addressed within the NHS (and social care) workforce by providing a comprehensive dataset that highlights the experiences of global majority staff (NHS Wales, 2024).

The 2024 NHS Wales Workforce Race Equality Standard report reveals notable differences to be addressed in leadership representation for staff from the global majority within NHS Wales. Despite making up 9.6% of the overall workforce, only 3.7% of senior leadership roles are held by the global majority staff. Put differently, while one in ten NHS employees are from minoritised backgrounds, just one in 30 board members reflect that diversity. Alarmingly, nine out of 13 NHS Wales organisations have no global majority representation at board level. These figures highlight the important need for targeted action to address structural areas for growth and ensure leadership pathways are equitable and inclusive.

In NHS Wales Health Boards, staff from the global majority often face areas for growth to career progression, with many becoming 'stuck' at Band 5. Representation drops significantly at higher bands, and one key contributing factor is the recruitment process. Data shows that, among shortlisted candidates, white applicants are 1.75 times more likely to be appointed than their global majority counterparts. While this may appear modest, the impact is cumulative. For example, a Band 5 nurse would need to secure eight successive promotions to reach Executive and Senior Post (ESP) level. Statistically, this means a White Band 5 nurse is 90 times more likely to reach ESP level than a global majority peer. The disparity is even more pronounced for Black nurses, where the likelihood increases to 420 times in favour of their White colleagues.

Further inequalities are evident in disciplinary and capability processes, where global majority nursing staff are disproportionately referred. These disparities vary across Health Boards, highlighting the need for consistent, fair, and transparent procedures.

The 2024 NHS Wales WRES report calls for data-driven action at the local level. One key recommendation is the introduction of a gateway review process for all disciplinary referrals—an independent, ideally executive-supervised mechanism to ensure fairness and eliminate racial bias, while maintaining patient safety as the highest priority.

For the nursing profession, these differences to be addressed have profound implications. They limit access to leadership opportunities, hinder professional growth, and adversely affect job satisfaction. Addressing these topics for enhancement is essential to building a diverse, inclusive nursing workforce that truly reflects and serves the communities of Wales.

The Nursing and Midwifery professions in Wales therefore have compelling reasons to drive improvement in the workforce data, and health outcomes of global majority populations. Evidence consistently shows inequities in care, particularly in maternity services. For example, Black pregnant women in the UK are more likely to receive poor-quality care, face disbelief when reporting pain, and are four times more likely to die during pregnancy or within six weeks postpartum compared to their White counterparts (MBRRACE-UK, 2021; 2023). These disparities stress the urgent need for anti-racist leadership and culturally competent care within nursing and midwifery.

Collective action is underway to shape a brighter, fairer future for the nursing and midwifery professions. This includes advancing workforce diversity, embedding cultural competence and anti-racist education, delivering equitable patient care, and cultivating inclusive work environments where every member of staff feels valued, supported, and empowered to thrive.

WRES Primary and Social Care Workforce

The 2024 WRES programme also produced inaugural reports for primary and social care staff, offering valuable insights into equity across the wider healthcare system. Using data from the Wales National Workforce and Reporting System (WNWRS) and the Workforce Inclusion and Belonging Survey, the report examined representation and experiences in pharmacy, dentistry, general practice, and optometry. It found that global majority staff make up 7.6% of the General Medical Services (GMS) workforce—broadly aligned with population demographics. However, only 1.6% of primary care decision-makers are from the global majority, despite high aspirations for progression. Alarmingly, global majority staff were over eight times more likely to report being referred into capability processes and over nine times more likely into disciplinary procedures compared to their White peers. Reports of bias—especially from colleagues and managers—were also significantly higher.

For nursing and midwifery, these findings reinforce the importance of embedding anti-racist principles across all sectors of care. They highlight the need to connect workforce equity with patient outcomes, ensuring that staff experiences inform service delivery. Translating this data into action requires Health Boards and Welsh Government to examine the systems and policies that perpetuate inequity—and to use their influence to disrupt them. Without this commitment, inequality will persist, and the vision of a truly inclusive and equitable Welsh healthcare system will remain unmet.

Improving Workforce Diversity in Nursing

Improving Representation

Workforce diversity is a central goal of the ARWAP, aiming to reflect the multicultural population of Wales. Historically, global majority individuals have been underrepresented in nursing leadership. To address this, targeted recruitment and retention initiatives have been introduced. For example, Swansea Bay University Health Board's Anti-Racist Workforce Action Plan includes strategies to attract diverse candidates, reduce bias in hiring, and create pathways for career progression (Swansea Bay University Health Board, 2022; 2024).

Advancing Leadership Opportunities

The ARWAP recognises that systemic barriers have historically limited global majority nurses' progression into senior roles. In response, leadership development programmes, mentorship schemes, and sponsorship initiatives have been introduced to support equitable career advancement. These efforts aim to prepare global majority nurses for senior positions and address longstanding underrepresentation. Sustained investment from the CNO has been key to ensuring these initiatives lead to lasting change.

The Aspiring Board Member Programme is one such strategic initiative launched by the Welsh Government and NHS Wales to address the notable underrepresentation of global majority individuals in senior leadership roles across the health system.

This programme is designed to equip global majority professionals with the skills, knowledge, and confidence to take up public appointments and board-level roles. Participants will gain a deeper understanding of the Welsh health system, develop leadership capabilities, and become 'board ready' for independent non-executive director positions.

Representation matters. Leadership that reflects the diversity of our workforce and communities is essential for building trust, driving equity, and delivering culturally competent care. By investing in the leadership potential of our global majority staff, we are not only correcting historical imbalances but also strengthening the future of our health service. This programme is an essential step toward dismantling systemic areas for growth, promoting inclusive governance, and ensuring that decision-making tables are enriched by diverse perspectives and lived experiences.

The programme which launched in 2025 is designed to support global majority individuals to secure and succeed in public appointments within health. Participants will bring relevant and valuable skills and experience. The programme will improve their understanding of the Welsh health system and help them recognise the value they can bring as leaders. By the end, there will be a cohort of Black, Asian, and minority ethnic individuals who are 'board ready' with new, valuable experience and knowledge specific to NHS Wales board contexts. Those individuals completing the course will be eligible to take up independent (non-executive) director positions on NHS Wales boards. To complement this, there needs to be talent development programmes in individual organisations to identify the clinical and non-clinical leaders of the future, so that a cadre of potential executive directors is identified.

Limitations of Top Tier Leadership

While initiatives like the Aspiring Board Member Programme represents a significant step forward, there is growing evidence—both in the UK and globally—that such top-tier leadership programmes often do not yet meet in delivering sustainable, systemic change for global majority staff.

Limited Structural Impact

A mixed-methods evaluation of the NHS Stepping Up and Ready Now programmes found that while participants valued the safe space and confidence-building aspects, the broader impact was constrained by ongoing institutional areas for growth and structural racism. Without parallel efforts to reform organisational culture and systems, leadership programmes possibility becoming aspirational rather than transformative (Blake et al., 2025).

Overemphasis on Individual Fixes

As far back as 2005 an essential review by the Health Foundation highlighted that many interventions focus on fixing the individual—through training, mentoring, or coaching—without addressing the organisational and cultural areas for growth that impede progression. This includes bias, need for access to informal networks, and developing exposure to high-impact roles (Esmail et al., 2005). In addition, such 'deficit model' approaches can create a culture of responsibility of the minoritised individual and diminish agency. As such interventions need to be incorporated alongside ones which tackle the root systemic causes and challenge privilege (Branova, 2023).

Neglect of Early-Career Pipeline

Global leadership programmes often concentrate on preparing individuals for board-level or executive roles, inadvertently overlooking the development of a diverse pipeline at junior and mid-career levels. This creates a narrow pathway where only a few are deemed 'ready' for top roles, while many talented individuals remain unsupported in their early progression.

Short-Termism and Lack of Continuity

Many programmes are time-limited and lack follow-up support, which can lead to a decline in momentum once the programme ends. Without longitudinal coaching or mentoring, participants may work hard to translate learning into tangible career advancement.

Global Lessons on Cultural Competence

Internationally, coaching models that embed cultural intelligence, intersectionality, and long-term support—such as those promoted by the International Coaching Federation—have shown greater promise. These models recognise that leadership development for global majority staff must be contextual, relational, and sustained over time (Straw, 2025).

Cultural Competency and Anti-Racism Training

The ARWAP prioritises cultural competency and anti-racism education. In response, the CNO has launched the national 'Getting to Equity' sponsorship programme to support aspiring global majority nurse and midwifery leaders, particularly those at Band 5 to 7. This reflects growing recognition that sustainable leadership requires early and mid-career development—not just top-tier programmes.

Nurses and midwives in NHS Wales also complete mandatory training to enhance cultural awareness and address unconscious bias, equipping them to deliver culturally sensitive care and recognise the social determinants of health affecting ethnic communities.

Undergraduate curricula are being revised to embed anti-racist principles, ensuring new graduates understand systemic racism and its impact on care delivery. In maternity services, all NHS Wales units have joined a cultural competency accreditation scheme supported by the Welsh Government, professional bodies, and unions. The four Higher Education Institutions (HEI)s responsible for pre-registration training are using the Royal College of Midwives' decolonising education toolkit to help educators create inclusive learning environments. The toolkit supports global majority students and addresses diverse maternity care needs through guidance on recruitment, curriculum, assessment, and practice (RCM, 2022).

Limitations of Cultural Competency Training

Cultural competency training often reduces 'culture' to race and ethnicity, overlooking other significant variables and identities such as gender, socioeconomic status, and disability. This reductionist approach can lead to generalisation and bias (Jongen et al., 2018).

In contrast, holistic approaches emphasise the interconnectedness and interdependence of parts within a system, viewing the whole as greater than the sum of its parts. This approach considers the relationships and interactions between components, rather than isolating and analysing individual parts.

Cultural competency training has faced criticism for its limited impact on systemic change. While widely implemented, such training often fails to address the deeper, structural causes of racism and inequality. Critics argue that it tends to focus on individual awareness rather than institutional reform. As a result, its effectiveness in improving equity and inclusion remains limited. To drive meaningful progress, a shift towards structural approaches—such as anti-racism strategies—is needed, targeting policies, systems, and workplace culture.

Anti-racism strategies are essential for fostering meaningful and lasting change. These approaches focus on reforming structural and institutional systems, policies, and processes, as well as addressing interpersonal racism—biases held by clinicians and staff—and internalised racism, which involves individuals from historically marginalised groups overcoming negative beliefs about their own worth and behaviours that sustain inequality (Vasan et al., 2024).

In summary, while cultural competency training aims to improve awareness and sensitivity, its limitations and the need for more systemic approaches make it a complex topic in the field of diversity and inclusion (Kamara, 2021). Recognising this, the Welsh Government—alongside the CNO—is actively developing to address deeper institutional inequalities.

Undergraduate Nursing Education and Anti-Racism Development in Wales

In Wales, undergraduate nursing education is a cornerstone of the healthcare workforce pipeline. Health Education and Improvement Wales (HEIW) commissions a wide range of nursing programmes across Welsh universities, including Adult, Child, Mental Health, and Learning Disability Nursing. These programmes are designed to meet the evolving needs of Health and Social Care Wales and are supported by full tuition funding and bursaries for eligible students.

Wales is investing in early-stage anti-racism education and leadership development, particularly through the work of HEIW, The Commission for Tertiary Education and Research (Medr), and the ARWAP.

HEIW plays a central role in shaping the future of the NHS workforce in Wales. Its education strategy prioritises:

- compassionate and inclusive leadership,
- equitable access to education and training,
- inter-professional learning, and
- Welsh language inclusion.

These principles are embedded in undergraduate and postgraduate training, helping to shape a culturally competent and diverse future workforce.

Medr has issued strategic guidance higher education in Wales. Its 2024/25 guidance includes:

- A requirement for all universities to achieve a Race Equality Charter award by 2025.
- Match funding for anti-racism initiatives.

- Monitoring of attainment opportunities.
- Support for emerging students to progress into employment or further study.

Limitations in Undergraduate Nursing Education and Anti-Racism Development in Wales

Despite a strong infrastructure, anti-racism development in undergraduate nursing education remains limited. While the ARWAP and Medr's 2024/25 guidance have set sector-wide expectations, most progress has focused on post-registration and senior leadership. Key initiatives include the Aspiring Board Member Programme, leadership schemes like Ready Now and Stepping Up, and organisational commitments to the Race Equality Charter. However, these efforts often overlook the foundational stage of professional identity—undergraduate education. Without early exposure to anti-racist principles, inclusive leadership, and culturally competent care, nursing and midwifery students may enter the workforce without the confidence or awareness needed to challenge systemic inequities.

Symbolic Progress vs. Structural Change

Professor Emmanuel Ogbonna reflects that while achieving the Advance HE Race Equality Charter Bronze Award is a positive step, it often signals institutional readiness rather than deep, embedded change. Without sustained commitment and cultural transformation, such recognition risks becoming symbolic rather than driving meaningful anti-racist reform (Ogbonna, 2024).

Short-Termism and Incentive Dependency

The success of Welsh universities in achieving bronze status was partly driven by funding requirements. While effective in the short term, this raises concerns about long-term sustainability—particularly if momentum fades without continued external pressure.

Overemphasis on Senior Roles

Critiques from the NHS and academic literature highlight a tendency to focus leadership development on board-level roles, often neglecting early-career professionals. This creates a narrow pathway where only a few are deemed 'ready', leaving many talented individuals unsupported.

Progress and Challenges

While progress has been made, challenges remain in translating the ARWAP's ambitions into consistent, measurable outcomes. Bridging the gap between policy and practice requires sustained investment in staffing, resources, and leadership development. For nursing and midwifery, this means embedding anti-racist principles into everyday practice and ensuring that equity is reflected in both workforce experiences and patient care. Continued advocacy is needed to uphold statutory duties under the Equality Act 2010 (UK Government, 2010) and the Well-being of Future Generations (Wales) Act 2015 (Welsh Government, 2025). With coordinated action and long-term commitment, the profession can help realise Wales's goal of becoming an anti-racist nation by 2030.

Conclusion

The ARWAP is a bold and progressive initiative that places nursing at the forefront of equity and transformation in healthcare.

Nursing leadership in Wales is driving meaningful change through inclusive governance, culturally competent care, and workforce diversity.

With continued commitment and collaboration, the profession is well-positioned to lead the way in creating a fairer, more inclusive health system for all.

Reflective Activity

Having read the chapter, we invite you to reflect on your key learning and its implications for your professional practice as a nurse or midwife using Bain et al.'s (2002) 5R framework (p. 13–15):

- Reporting—What is it in your situation you want to transform after reading this chapter?
- Responding—What are your personal observations regarding your own situation/context in relation to what is raised in this chapter?
- Relating—What is/are the theoretical/research/data/legislative, etc., understandings relationship to under consideration in this chapter that you could apply to your situation/context?
- Reasoning—Identify how the chapter findings matter to your situation/context and how will you interrogate your situation/context and what will help you from this chapter?
- Reconstructing—Identify your action plans to reframe and rebuild a transformative way forward to change from the situation in your context.

References

Bain, J.D., Ballantyne, R., Mills, C. and Lester, N.C. (2002). *Reflecting on practice: Students teachers' perspectives*. Post Pressed.

Blake, H., Scarlett, K., Khulumula, S.K. and Chouliara, N. (2025). Mixed-methods evaluation of targeted leadership development training to support the career progression of the black and minority ethnic NHS workforce. *BMJ Leader*. https://doi.org/10.1136/leader-2024-001175

Branova, S. (2023). *The asset model: An approach to teaching and education*. American Society for Microbiology. https://asm.org/articles/2023/december/the-asset-model-an-approach-to-teaching-and-educat

Cummings, J. and Serrant, L. (2018). *BME nurses and midwives instrumental in helping shape the NHS of today*.

Dahl, K., Nortvedt, L., Schrøder, J. and Bjørnnes, A.K. (2022). Internationally educated nurses and resilience: A systematic literature review. *International Nursing Review*, *69*(4), 512–524. https://doi.org/10.1111/inr.12787

Di Iasio, V., Giulietti, C. and Wahba, J. (2024). *Mind the opportunity: Education, employment and mobility of second-generation immigrants in the UK*. Centre for Population Change. Policy Briefing No. 75. https://www.cpc.ac.uk/docs/PB75_Mind_the_gap_Education_employment_and_mobility_of_second-generation_immigrants_in_the_UK.pdf

Dustmann, C., Frattini, T. and Theodoropoulos, N. (2010). *Ethnicity and second generation immigrants in Britain, CReAM Discussion Paper Series, No. 04/10*. Centre for Research and Analysis of Migration (CReAM), Department of Economics, University College London. https://www.econstor.eu/bitstream/10419/295350/1/cream-dp1004.pdf

Esmail, A., Lalra, V. and Abel, P. (2005). *Ethnic minority patients' experiences of the NHS: An essential review of the literature*. University of Manchester.

Francis, R. (2013). *Report of the mid Staffordshire NHS foundation trust public inquiry*. The Stationery Office. https://www.gov.uk/government/publications/report-of-the-mid-staffordshire-nhs-foundation-trust-public-inquiry

Kamara, K. (2021). *Using an anti-racist approach to address patient social needs*. Leonard Davis Institute of Health Economics.

Kapadia, D., Zhang, J., Salway, S., Nazroo, J., Booth, A., Villarroel-Williams, N., Becares, L. and Esmail, A. (2022). *Ethnic inequalities in healthcare: A rapid review*. NHS Race & Health Observatory. https://www.nhsrho.org/wp-content/uploads/2023/05/RHO-Rapid-Review-Final-Report_.pdf

Kapilashrami, A., Otis, M., Omodara, D., Nandi, A., Vats, A., Adeniyi, O., Speed, E., Potter, J.L., Eder, B., Pareek, M., Bhui, K. and the I-COPE Consortium. (2022). Ethnic disparities in health & social care workers' exposure, protection, and clinical management of the COVID-19 pandemic in the UK. *Critical Public Health*, *32*(1), 68–81. https://doi.org/10.1080/09581596.2021.1959020

Lanada, J.A. and Culligan, K. (2024). The experiences of internationally educated nurses who joined the nursing workforce in England. *British Journal of Nursing*, *33*(2), 78–84. https://doi.org/10.12968/bjon.2024.33.2.78

Mashinkila, W., Bosun-Arije, S. and Heyes, K. (2023). An insight into the experiences of Black and minority ethnic nurses within healthcare: A narrative literature review. *International Journal of Advanced Nursing Education and Research*, *8*(1), 33–44. http://dx.doi.org/10.21742/ijaner.2023.8.1.03

MBRRACE-UK. (2021). Disparity in maternal deaths because of ethnicity is "unacceptable". *BMJ*, *372*, n152. https://doi.org/10.1136/bmj.n152

MBRRACE-UK. (2023). Maternal mortality rates in the UK. https://www.npeu.ox.ac.uk/assets/downloads/mbrrace-uk/reports/maternal-report-2023/MBRRACE-UK_Maternal_Compiled_Report_2023.pdf

NHS Confederation. (2022). The unequal impact of COVID-19: Investigating the effect on people with certain protected characteristics. https://www.nhsconfed.org/publications/unequal-impact-covid-19-protected-characteristics

NHS England. (2021). *Action required to tackle health inequalities in latest phase of COVID-19 response and recovery*. https://www.england.nhs.uk/about/equality/equality-hub/national-healthcare-inequalities-improvement-programme/what-are-healthcare-inequalities/action-required-to-tackle-health-inequalities-in-latest-phase-of-covid-19-response-and-recovery/

NHS England. (2024). *Workforce Race Equality Standard (WRES) annual report 2024*. NHS England.

NHS Wales. (2024). *National Workforce Race Equality Standard (WRES) report 2024*. NHS Wales.

NHS Wales Shared Services Partnership. (2023). *All Wales International Recruitment Programme 2022*. https://performanceandimprovement.nhs.wales/functions/quality-safety-and-improvement/improvement/nhs-wales-awards/2024/workforce-sustainability/nwssp-recruitment-programme/#:~:text=Commissioned%20by%20the%20Welsh%20Government%20in%202021%2C%20the,offers%20were%20made%2C%20achieving%2097%25%20of%20the%20target

NIHR Evidence. (2022). *Healthcare workers from ethnic minorities felt unsafe during the pandemic*. National Institute for Health and Care Research.

Nursing and Midwifery Counci (NMC). (2025). *Wales data report: March 2025*. Nursing and Midwifery Council.

Office for National Statistics. (2022). *Ethnic group, national identity, language and religion in Wales: Census 2021*. https://www.gov.wales/ethnic-group-national-identity-language-and-religion-wales-census-2021-html

Ogbonna, E. (2024). *Race equality charter success for Welsh HE Institutions*. Advance HE.

Peate, I. (2024). International recruitment. *British Journal of Nursing*, *33*(7), 23–325. https://doi.org/10.12968/bjon.2024.33.7.323

Race Disparity Unit, Equality Hub. (2023). *Outcomes in labour market for ethnic minorities by immigrant generation status*. GOV.UK.

Rhead, R., Harber-Aschan, L., Onwumere, J., Polling, C., Dorrington, S., Ehsan, A., Stevelink, S.A.M., Khunti, K., Mir, G., Morriss, R., Wessely, S., Woodhead, C. and Hatch, S. (2024). Ethnic inequalities among NHS staff in England: Workplace experiences during the COVID-19 pandemic. *Occupational & Environmental Medicine*, *81*(3), 13–121. https://doi.org/10.1136/oemed-2023-108976

RJongen, C., McCalman, J. and Bainbridge, R. (2018). Health workforce cultural competency interventions: A systematic scoping review. *BMC Health Services Research*, *18*(1), 232. https://doi.org/10.1186/s12913-018-3001-5

Royal College of Midwives. (2022). *Decolonising Midwifery Education Toolkit*. https://rcm.org.uk/publications/decolonising-midwifery-education-toolkit/

Sanches, D., Pereira, S., Castro, S., Mendes, M., Santos, E. and Ribeiro, O. (2024). Generational diversity in nursing practice environments: Scoping review. *BMC Nursing*, *23*, 928. https://doi.org/10.1186/s12912-024-02607-3

Straw, M. (2025). *The opportunities and possibilities of global leadership programmes and how to overcome them*. Achieve Breakthrough.

Swansea Bay University Health Board. (2022). *Workforce Anti-Racist Action Plan*. sbuhb.nhs.wales/about-us/key-documents-folder/workforce-and-od-committee-papers/workforce-and-od-committee-october-2022/24-appendix-apdf/

Swansea Bay University Health Board. (2024). *People Strategy 2024–2029*. sbuhb.nhs.wales/about-us/key-documents-folder/workforce-and-od-committee-papers/workforce-and-od-committee-february-2024/7-2-appendix-1-people-strategy-pdf/

Tamburello, H., Maynard, E., Tse, J., Campbell, M., Burnham, J. and Argyrides, A. (2025). *Unreciprocated care: Why internationally educated nursing staff are leaving the UK*. Royal College of Nursing.

UK Government. (2010). Equality Act 2010, c.15. https://www.gov.uk/guidance/equality-act-2010-guidance

Vasan, A., Dalembert, G. and Garg, A. (2024). An anti-racist approach to social care integration. *Pediatrics*, *153*(1), e2023062109. https://doi.org/10.1542/peds.2023-062109

Welsh Government. (2022). *Anti-Racist Wales Action Plan*. Welsh Government.

Welsh Government. (2022). *Chief Nursing Officer for Wales: Priorities 2022 to 2024*. Welsh Government.

Welsh Government. (2023). *National Workforce Implementation Plan: Addressing NHS Wales Workforce Challenges*. Welsh Government.

Welsh Government. (2025). Well-being of Future Generations (Wales) Act 2015.

West, E. and Nayar, S. (2016). *A review of the literature on the experiences of Black, minority and internationally recruited nurses and midwives in the UK healthcare system*. Nursing and Midwifery Council.

8

RACISM AND HEALTH INEQUITY

A Nursing and Midwifery Perspective from Brazil

Patricia Lima Ferreira Santa Rosa, Rafaella Pires Vieira, and Nathalya Fonseca Camargo

Introduction

Childbirth care in Brazil has historically been traversed by structural inequalities that reflect processes of exclusion (Leal et al., 2017), among them Obstetric Racism (OR) (Davis, 2019). In this context, understanding the trajectory of childbirth care in the country requires a critical analysis of care and institutional practices, professional training, social participation, and public policies (Leite et al., 2022), highlighting the need for anti-racism care that values diverse forms of knowledge and promotes equity in the assistance provided to Black women (BW) (Rebouças et al., 2024).

To better understand the obstetric landscape in Brazil, it is relevant to examine statistical data on maternal and child health care. For context, the Brazilian population is composed of a majority of Black people, divided between *pretas* (dark-skinned Black) and *pardas* (Brown or mixed-heritage), who together account for 56% of the population (IBGE – Brazilian Institute of Geography and Statistics, 2022). In this regard, a recent study showed that the maternal mortality rate in the country is higher among BW compared to White women (Coelho et al., 2022). Moreover, BW exhibit other indicators that reveal racial disparities, such as a higher likelihood of inadequate prenatal care, higher prevalence of post-term births (gestational period exceeding 41 completed weeks), lack of prior linkage to a maternity hospital, absence of a birth companion, and greater need to move between health facilities during labour (Leal et al., 2017). Although episiotomy is not an evidence-based practice and can sometimes be classified as obstetric violence (OV) (Fiocruz, 2023) (Fiocruz is at the forefront of Brazil's public health strategy, including scientific rigour with need for social equity), the disparity here is that BW receive less local anaesthesia when the procedure is performed (Leal et al., 2022).

DOI: 10.4324/9781003565369-8

With respect to childbirth care professionals, there are four categories: traditional midwives (TM), midwives, nurse-midwives (NM), and obstetric physicians, each with distinct training, practices, and institutional placement (Souza, 2023). Historically, childbirth was first assisted by TM, who provided family and home-based care, grounded in knowledge handed down through the generations. Over time, childbirth underwent a transition that culminated in more biomedical and hospital-centred care. Today, TM primarily serves rural, riverside, and *quilombola* (African-Brazilian people remaining from *quilombo*) communities (Souza, 2023). In Brazil, midwives are professionals trained in midwives school at the University of São Paulo since 2005. Their model of care emphasises the humanisation of childbirth, prioritizing the autonomy and centring of those who gestate and give birth (Koga, 2022), while facing numerous challenges in a still hegemonically biomedical system (Souza, 2023). Nurse-midwives must complete a nursing degree followed by postgraduate training in obstetrics. Their education tends to be biologically oriented, though with a growing trend towards humanized care (Araújo et al., 2019). Obstetric physicians complete a medical degree followed by residency in obstetrics and gynaecology. They currently dominate in childbirth care (Souza, 2023). Traditionally, the obstetrics and gynaecology profession follows a hospital-centred model that often reinforces medicalized interventionist practices (Souza, 2023), which disproportionately affect BW (Leal et al., 2017).

OR operates within institutional and structural spheres, arising from the intersection of OV and medical racism (Davis, 2019). OV is a form of institutional and gender-based violence occurring during pregnancy, childbirth, postpartum, and abortion, manifesting in health services, particularly in contexts of heightened vulnerability (Zanardo et al., 2017). This violence may be expressed through disrespectful attitudes, offensive language, abuse of authority, omission of care, and inappropriate physical interventions (Fiocruz, 2023). Medical racism extends beyond physicians, involving the entire team of health professionals engaged in obstetric care (Tempesta & Eneile, 2021). It is evident from differences in clinical practices, therapeutic choices, diagnostic approaches, and overall quality of care provided to Black patients, resulting in negative health and safety outcomes (Davis, 2019).

Nurse-midwives and midwives, whose training is rooted comprehensively in biomedical care and health equity, hold a strategic position to confront OR (Costa et al., 2024). Racism, however, is embedded stubbornly in systems and hence requires collective efforts, across professions and health and social care institutes, to be dismantled (Silva et al., 2023). In obstetrics, these efforts span health care, management, and education.

Still, nurse-midwives (NM) and midwives face significant challenges in developing anti-racist practice. First, professional training is largely bio-medical focussed, neglecting interdisciplinary and cultural approaches. Hospital-centred models prioritize protocols and traditional medical practices, often leading to non-evidence-based interventions and iatrogenic outcomes. Second, the widely diffused "myth of racial democracy" (Fernandes, 1972) sustains the notion of racial harmony and equal opportunity, denying the existence and consequences of systemic and institutional racism. This fallacy of "racial democracy" obscures the specific health needs of the Black population (Anunciação et al., 2022). Third, universities struggle to comply with Resolution No. 569 (2017), which mandates that health programs address ethnic-racial relations, African-Brazilian and African culture, and the differences in traditional communities and human rights (National Health Council, 2017).

The History and Context of Obstetric Care in Brazil

Childbirth care in Brazil has a long trajectory, from the colonial period to the contemporary model. Initially, TM were responsible for births from colonization until the mid-nineteenth century (Souza, 2023). Today, they remain important for riverside, quilombola, and rural communities, offering family- and home-based care. Hospital births began in the late-nineteenth century but only became widespread in the mid-twentieth century. Until the 1960s, most Brazilians were born at home with midwives' assistance (Palharini & Figueirôa, 2018). Historically, TM played a central role in childbirth, sharing popular knowledge and empirical practices across generations (Souza, 2023).

Biomedical advances and the institutionalization of care, especially with the rise of hospitals and medical schools, shifted childbirth towards a physician-centred model (Carraca Pitta et al., 2024). While advances in disease prevention, obstetric risk management, and evidence-based techniques were undeniable, this transition marginalized TM and concentrated care under formally trained professionals, increasing unnecessary interventions (Souza, 2023). Brazil's caesarean section rates exemplify this: exceeding 80% in private hospitals (Brazil, ANS, 2023) compared to the World Health Organization's recommendation of 10–15% (WHO, 2015).

The Health System in Brazil

Brazil's health system is mixed, composed of public and private sectors. The Unified Health System (SUS – abbreviation in Portuguese), the public healthcare system, established by the 1988 Federal Constitution, is grounded in universality, integrality, and equity, guaranteeing free and comprehensive health care for all residents, including immigrants and refugees (Brazil, 1990). The private sector plays a complementary role, accessible primarily through insurance or direct payment (Brazil, 1998). Despite the availability of private services, the SUS is the main pathway to care, serving about 80% of the population (Brazil, Ministry of Health, 2021), which exceeds 210 million people (Brazil, IBGE, 2024). It is estimated that 67% of SUS users are Black (Paixão et al., 2010). Key programs include the National Immunization Program (PNI), which ensures free vaccination (Brazil, Ministry of Health, 1975); the Mobile Emergency Care Service (SAMU), which provides free 24/7 emergency care to 85% of the population (Brazil, Ministry of

Health, 2022); and the National Health Surveillance Agency (ANVISA – abbreviation in Portuguese), responsible for regulating food, cosmetics, medicines, and vaccines (Brazil, Ministry of Health, n.d.).

The SUS is the largest public healthcare system in the world, in terms of both the scope of services provided and the population covered (Brazil, Ministry of Health, 2022). Care is organized by levels of complexity, in order to ensure the integrality of care, beginning with Primary Health Care, the entry point and encompasses low-complexity services with broad capillarity, focused on promotion, prevention, and continuity of care. In maternal health, pregnant women are monitored in Basic Health Units and Family Health Strategies. In this context, they are followed up by general practitioners and nurses, receiving prenatal care, counselling, vaccines, and routine examinations, such as physical and obstetric assessments, as well as basic prenatal tests and exams, including obstetric ultrasounds (Brazil, Ministry of Health, 2011a).

Peri-hospital Normal Birth Centres (BC), popularly known as birthing centres, also operate at primary and secondary care levels. They provide prenatal and postpartum visits, health education, and usual-risk childbirth care. These units were officially regulated in Brazil in 1999 (Brazil, Ministry of Health, 1999). Currently, 13 centres operate nationwide. BC are intended to provide care for women and newborns at usual risk, so care is provided by midwives and NM, with no physician required on staff (Brazil, Ministry of Health, 1999); a point of tension in Brazil's biomedical culture (Aguiar et al., 2025). Evidence indicates that this model of care is associated with an increase in the occurrence of vaginal births and improved childbirth experiences, as well as with a reduction in the incidence of instrumental vaginal deliveries, preterm births (<37 weeks), and foetal or neonatal deaths, thus demonstrating the safety of this type of obstetric care (Carregal et al., 2020).

Specialized healthcare is organized into two subgroups: secondary and tertiary levels. Secondary care, in turn, encompasses specialized medium-complexity services, such as Emergency Care Units, serving as a complement to primary healthcare units. This level of care includes specialty outpatient clinics and referral centres (Brazil, Ministry of Health, 2022), such as high-risk prenatal outpatient services and reference centres for pregnant women with comorbidities. In these facilities, additional examinations, such as specialized ultrasounds, as well as follow-up by obstetricians, are provided to ensure maternal-foetal safety. Furthermore, secondary care also involves some medium-complexity maternity hospitals, where certain types of vaginal births are performed (Brazil, Ministry of Health, 2023a) and may be attended by midwives, nurse-midwives, and obstetricians (Fiocruz, 2019). Tertiary care, meanwhile, involves high-complexity services aimed at cases requiring hospitalization and specialized procedures, such as maternity hospitals and referral hospitals (Brazil, Ministry of Health, 2022). These facilities provide certain types of vaginal births, caesarean sections, and admissions to neonatal or adult intensive care units (ICUs) when necessary. This level ensures advanced support for obstetric complications, such as HELLP syndrome, as well as infrastructure support for extremely preterm newborns (gestational age < 28 weeks) (Brazil, Ministry of Health, 2014; 2023a). Midwives and nurse-midwives may also assist in normal low-risk deliveries, while obstetricians are responsible for high-risk vaginal births, caesarean sections, and certain ICU care (Fiocruz, 2019). Thus, the SUS organises maternal healthcare in a hierarchical and integrated manner, aiming to ensure comprehensive and efficient care throughout all stages of pregnancy, childbirth, and the postpartum.

Despite the advances and benefits associated with the medicalization of childbirth and birth, the hospitalization of this process has also led to the adoption of unnecessary interventions, contributing to the emergence and consolidation of the phenomenon of OV (Souza, 2023). Childbirth, previously understood as part of the female experience, came to be regarded as a male-dominated medical experience, in which the notion of childbirth as a high-risk event became the norm rather than the exception. This has resulted in a reduction of the agency and autonomy of birthing individuals, as well as the institutionalization of their bodies (Zanardo et al., 2017). This context has also deepened historical inequalities, culminating in racialized OR (Davis, 2019).

Obstetric Racism: Concept, Impact, and Consequences

OR emerges from the intersectionality of OV and medical racism (Davis, 2019). Recognized for coining the term, anthropologist Dána-Ain Davis is currently a professor at Queens College, City University of New York, United States. Her writings focus on the intersections of race and reproductive health, particularly in the US context (American Anthropological Association, 2023). Davis has made significant contributions to the consolidation of the concept of OR, whose influence has expanded beyond the United States and become a reference in global debates on racial inequities in obstetric care.

OV is a form of gender-based and institutional violence that occurs throughout the reproductive cycle—during pregnancy, childbirth, postpartum, or abortion—particularly in health care environments where women are vulnerable. This violence may manifest through humiliating behaviours, abuse of authority, neglect, and physical violations, among others (Zanardo et al., 2017). Medical racism, in this context, refers not only to physicians' actions but to all health professionals engaged in obstetric care (Tempesta & Eneile, 2021). It is characterized by differential treatment, diagnosis, and clinical conduct based on race, directly shaping care decisions and placing BW at higher risk (Davis, 2019). Its origins lie in misguided historical conceptions of Black bodies, perpetuated by racial stereotypes and remnants of social hierarchies from slavery (Davis, 2020).

Although the concept of OR was formalized in 2018 (Davis, 2018), racial disparities in maternal health had long been observed in Brazil (Brazil, Ministry of Health, 2023b). The emergence of the term "obstetric racism" is important given the complexity of the phenomenon, in which racism structures and amplifies gender-based violence. Thus, the isolated definitions of OV and medical racism are insufficient to encompass its totality in maternal health (Davis, 2019). The adoption of the concept of OR serves as a political communication strategy to prevent the naturalization or erasure of the fact that BW are the primary victims of violent and negligent practices during pregnancy, childbirth, postpartum, and abortion (Rodrigues, 2020).

As an example, consider the case of Maria – a fictitious name for a Black Brazilian woman – whose childbirth experiences were marked by OR. In her first labour, she wore *box-braids*, but significant decelerations in foetal heart rate required an emergency caesarean. During preparation for surgery, the obstetrician in charge ordered the immediate removal of her braids – a practice unfortunately common in Brazil – under the pretext of preventing burns from electrocautery. Given the time required to remove *box-braids* and the need for immediate intervention that Maria's child required, this conduct alone would already be considered highly negligent. Worse still, this order was carried out through yelling, coercion, and the humiliation of Maria, treating her as irresponsible and endangering her baby simply for wearing braids.

In her second labour, Maria arrived at the hospital in active labour – with strong, regular contractions and advanced cervical dilation – seeking care due to intense pain. Upon arrival, however, her complaints were completely ignored. Moreover, the nurse-midwife caring for her neither offered available non-pharmacological pain relief methods (such as a warm shower or massage by her companion) nor acknowledged her suffering. Instead, she told Maria that she was weak, adding that women like her – that is, BW – were supposed to be stronger and more resistant to pain.

Maria's case, unfortunately based on real events, illustrates how OR operates in practice. Davis identifies dimensions of OR that include critical diagnostic delays, negligent conduct, humiliating treatment, intentional infliction of pain, limited pain relief options, coercion into procedures, degrading situations, abuse of power, and the pervasive fear of encountering racism in the health system. In Maria's story, multiple dimensions of OR acted simultaneously, intensifying the violence. OR represents a threat not only to women's health but also to newborns, compromising maternal and neonatal outcomes in the Black population (Davis, 2019).

Moreover, narratives from BW frequently reveal experiences of silencing by physicians, exposing the persistence of authoritarian conduct, disregard for their expressions of pain and suffering, and frequent violations of legally guaranteed rights. Far from isolated cases, these practices reflect the reproduction of a hierarchical top-down model of care that ignores ethno-racial specificities and sustains inequalities in obstetric care (Lima et al., 2021). Maternal mortality among BW thus constitutes both a grave public health problem and a violation of women's human and reproductive rights (Bessa et al., 2023). OR is a systemic reality in Brazil's health care system, directly affecting indicators such as maternal mortality and maternal near miss (Brazil, Ministry of Health, 2023c). It also negatively influences childbirth experiences: BW report greater dissatisfaction with obstetric care compared to White women, which affects their entire journey of gestating, birthing, and mothering (Santos et al., 2024).

OR also deeply shapes experiences of abortion, it profoundly impacts women's experiences regarding the abortion process, from unplanned pregnancy to the decision for interruption. Frequently, they must make this decision without emotional, socioeconomic, and institutional support networks, intensifying vulnerabilities imposed by structural inequalities (Goes, 2023). Racial disparities in obstetric indicators are evident throughout the reproductive cycle of BW. Studies show higher risks of inadequate prenatal care, post-term births, absence of linkage to a maternity hospital, lack of a birth companion, and "peregrination" in search of care during labour, compared to White women (Leal et al., 2017). OR is a severe public health problem with direct impacts on maternal morbidity and mortality among BW. Confronting these practices requires effective actions grounded in principles of anti-racism, equity, and human rights. NM and midwives have a strategic role in advancing anti-racist care, the focus of the next part of this chapter.

Obstetric Anti-Racism: Nurse-Midwives and Midwives

Although the Black population constitutes the proportional majority of Brazilian society (IBGE, 2022) and also makes up the majority of users of the SUS (Paixão et al., 2010), research and health care has historically failed to adequately address issues related to racialisation/racism. Understanding OR is essential to reveal the magnitude of the problem, which threatens not only the health and well-being of BW but also their access to disease prevention and health promotion (Tempesta & Eneile, 2021). According to the Epidemiological Report – Health of the Black Population – Volume 1, more than 90% of maternal deaths caused by direct obstetric factors are preventable (Brazil, Ministry of Health, 2023b). This is particularly true when there is timely access to health services, especially prenatal care (Brazil, Ministry of Health, 2009).

In recent decades, Brazil has made significant strides in addressing health inequalities, particularly those affecting vulnerable populations. Among the most relevant initiatives are the creation of the SUS in 1990 (Brazil, Ministry of Health, 1990) and the implementation of the Comprehensive Health Care on Women Health: Principles and directives (PNAISM – abbreviation in Portuguese) in 2004 (Brazil, Ministry of Health, 2011b). Specifically regarding the Black population, the formulation of the PNSIPN in 2010 deserves special mention (Brazil, Ministry of Health, 2016). Despite these achievements, numerous challenges persist. In urgent anti-racism response for healthcare in Brazil, Resolution No. 569 was enacted in 2017. Its aim was the defence of life, of the SUS, and of the fulfilment of social health needs, including aspects related to racialisation and ethnicity (National Health Council, 2017). For nursing professionals, including NM and midwives, there is a draft resolution proposing an update to the National Curriculum Guideline;

focusing on generalist, critical, reflective, political, and ethical training in order to strengthen the profession and improve the quality of health care provided to the Black population (Higher Education Chamber of the National Council of Education, 2024).

To give some context, the nursing workforce in Brazil is largely composed of BW. According to the Federal Nursing Council (COFEN – abbreviation in Portuguese), the workforce is predominantly female, with a large proportion self-identifying as Black – especially at the technical and auxiliary levels, without a university degree (Fiocruz & COFEN, 2017). They occupy roles mostly as nursing technicians and assistants, and some are nurses, revealing the intersections of racialisation/ethnicity, identity, gender, and class in the division of labour in health care. This configuration demonstrates how obstetric care, despite being central to public health, remains structured by inequalities that position BW at the base of the professional hierarchy (Akotirene, 2018). As Crenshaw emphasises, it is precisely in the overlapping of oppressions that the political and transformative potential for healthcare change can occur for BW (Crenshaw, 2002). However evidence-informed midwifery and NM, contributes to improved health indicators while upholding the autonomy and centring women in their care across health care and the pregnancy-birth-postpartum period (Souza, 2023). These aspects directly foster the humanization of childbirth and birth and promote equitable and anti-racist care (Lima et al., 2021).

Practicing according to ethical and humanizing good practice in obstetric care and health equity is crucial for anti-racism change across nursing; helping reduce racial disparities and inequities (Costa et al., 2024). Midwives and NM can strengthen their care network by valuing TM's ancestral knowledge and promoting integration between traditional practices and modern evidence-based approaches (Souza, 2023). Strengthening and valuing these TM professionals are fundamental strategies to ensure the promotion of human rights, particularly those of women and newborns, and to expand access to quality reproductive care in quilombola and rural communities. Recognizing TMs' roles in childbirth, birth, and reproductive planning contributes to the construction of more humanized health services (Souza, 2023). Their contribution extends beyond sensitive clinical interventions, encompassing political engagement in health care networks, the training of new professionals, and community mobilisation to advance racial equity and the reproductive sovereignty of BW.

In the field of education, nurse educators can adopt an ethical-political anti-racism stance in pedagogies, shaping the training of professionals committed to reducing racial inequities in health. This may involve incorporating racial literacy as a fundamental element in confronting racism. Yet, many challenges persist in implementing anti-racism measures in nursing and midwifery training, demanding continuous efforts in curricular review, faculty training, and the strengthening of equity inclusive educational policies (Souza et al., 2024). Importantly, anti-racist actions must not remain confined to theory. To be effectively enacted, they must reach praxis. Theory provides the foundation for practice, but tangible results cannot be achieved by remaining solely at the theoretical level (bell hooks, 1994). Anti-racist training will embed and operationalise when health is recognized as racist and professionals are prepared to act with social responsibility in the face of unjust structural inequalities.

Training health professionals with an anti-racism focus has been associated with reductions in disparities, improvements in quality of care, enhanced patient experiences, and, consequently, better health outcomes – such as reductions in maternal morbidity and mortality (Leal et al., 2017). Addressing race-related issues also strengthens the SUS, aligning with its core principles of effective evidence-informed care and equity, while reinforcing the objectives of the Comprehensive Health Care National Policy of Negro Population: an Unified Health Sistem Policy (SUS – Brazil) (PNSIPN – abbreviation in Portuguese) (Brazil, Ministry of Health, 2016). At the managerial level, the anti-racist role of health managers can shape both local health units and the formulation and implementation of public policies aimed at racial equity in care (Werneck, 2016). After all they are in a power position to facilitate change. This requires collaboration with social movements, professional councils, and government bodies to ensure that combating racism is firmly embedded in the public health agenda (Brazil, Ministry of Health, 2016).

The following highlights ongoing initiatives in Brazil addressing OR: the *Alyne Network Program*, the *Little Guide to Obstetric Anti-Racism*, and the Maternal Mortality among Black women: a workshop report in the Brazilian Health System context.

Alyne Network Program

The program is named in honour of Alyne Pimentel, a Black woman who died in 2002, losing her baby at six months of gestation, as a result of negligence and omission of obstetric care (Brazil, Ministry of Health, 2024b). Her case led to Brazil being condemned by an international court—the first judgment worldwide to recognize a preventable maternal death as a grave violation of human rights, specifically the right to safe motherhood (National Health Council, 2024).

Established in 2024, the Alyne Network Program (*Rede Alyne in Portuguese)* is a federal public program that replaced the previous Stork Network Program (*Rede Cegonha in Portuguese*), incorporating a set of governmental measures aimed at reducing maternal mortality in Brazil (Brazil, Ministry of Health, 2024a). The program sets two primary goals: to reduce overall maternal mortality by 25% and maternal mortality among BW by 50% (National Health Council, 2024). It promotes the expansion of humanized, comprehensive care for pregnant, birthing, and postpartum women and for children, taking into account specificities and vulnerabilities.

The program provides new funding to improve the quality and safety of primary health care, with emphasis on access to reproductive planning and appropriate prenatal care for women at usual obstetric risk. It also calls for restructuring obstetric emergency services to eliminate the so-called "pilgrimage" of women seeking care during labour. Furthermore, it includes strategies to promote breastfeeding, including expanding the supply of human milk in neonatal units (Brazil, Ministry of Health, 2024a).

The Alyne Network Program represents a significant step in addressing OR and reducing health inequities, particularly maternal mortality among BW (Brazil, Ministry of Health, 2024b). The initiative reflects recognition by the State of the urgent need for professional practice attuned to identifying and confronting ethno-racial inequalities that negatively impact maternal and neonatal outcomes. It underscores the importance of obstetric care that is sensitive to racial specificities, committed to equity, and grounded in human rights principles. Additionally, it highlights the central role NM and midwives play in confronting OR, by explicitly prioritizing their leadership in obstetric care (Brazil, Ministry of Health, 2024a).

The Little Guide to Obstetric Anti-Racism

The *Little Guide to Obstetric Anti-Racism* (Ferreira, 2023) provides well-grounded recommendations intended to equip pregnant women and their families to recognize and address manifestations of OR. Its guidance applies to both public and private health services (Agência de Notícias das Favelas, Favelas News Agency, 2024). The guide was developed in 2023 by the working group on OR coordinated by Rio de Janeiro city councilwoman Thais Ferreira (Ferreira, 2023).

The guide defines and contextualizes OR, presenting associated factors that shape its occurrence and offering a legislative overview in Brazil. It focuses on identifying forms of obstetric care during prenatal visits, childbirth, and postpartum that are permeated by OR, with the aim of raising awareness among pregnant and birthing women and their support networks to prevent violent and discriminatory practices in reproductive health care. In addition, it provides educational strategies for confronting OR on an individual level, emphasizing the importance of reporting such cases as a means of ensuring professional and institutional accountability and advancing reproductive justice (Agência de Notícias das Favelas, Favelas News Agency, 2024; Ferreira, 2023).

Maternal Mortality among Black Women: A Workshop Report in the Brazilian Health System Context

The *Maternal Mortality among Black Women: A Workshop Report in the Brazilian Health System Context* is an initiative of the Brazilian Ministry of Health aimed at tackling OR and maternal mortality among BW. Its primary objectives include promotion of institutional coordination for the strengthening of strategies addressing the social determinants of maternal mortality among BW. The report proposes the training of SUS professionals to confront racism, one of the main factors driving this scenario. It also seeks to support the formulation of actions to consolidate and expand both the PNAISM and the PNSIPN, taking into account local and regional specificities. Moreover, it emphasises the dissemination of knowledge and practices through dialogue among researchers, health professionals, managers, Black faculty, students, and the general population, integrated into the training of human resources within the SUS (Brazil, Ministry of Health, 2025).

The final report also includes maternal health indicators such as maternal mortality, morbidity, and maternal near miss, while discussing sociodemographic, obstetric, and equity-related issues (Brazil, Ministry of Health, 2025).

Conclusion

Confronting racism in obstetrics in Brazil requires a collective and coordinated commitment to anti-racism transformation, that goes beyond traditional clinical care settings, integrating education, professional training, and structural public policies. Anti-racist education must be understood as a continuous and collaborative designed and coproduced process involving not only pregnant women but also health professionals – especially NM, midwives, obstetricians, nursing technicians, and assistants – as well as health systems managers. Healthcare guided by obstetric anti-racism must promote practices centred on respecting the autonomy of BW, valuing their ancestral knowledge and subjective experiences, which have historically been rendered invisible, devalued, or delegitimized. This requires profound transformations in models of care, breaking with excessive medicalization and institutional violence, while ensuring access to humanized, comprehensive, and culturally sensitive care (Akotirene, 2018).

From the perspective of public policy, it is crucial that obstetric anti-racism be incorporated transversally into governmental agendas, involving the Ministry of Health, and the Secretariats of Education, Human Rights, and Racial Equality. Strengthening the PNSIPN (Brazil, Ministry of Health, 2016) must be accompanied by specific funding for training, monitoring, and combating institutional racism within maternal and child health services. Equally important is the active participation of BW and social movements, who have historically led efforts to denounce OV and propose community-based solutions such as support groups, networks of doulas, TM, and spaces for listening and political education (Gonzalez, 2020; Ribeiro, 2017). Institutional recognition and support for these grassroots initiatives are essential to legitimize and expand practices that have already proven effective in confronting racism and promoting reproductive health.

Although the Brazilian context has its own cultural and historical specificities, lessons drawn from local experiences and anti-racist practices in obstetrics can contribute to the global debate on reproductive justice and health equity. The pursuit of health systems that are more just, equitable, and fully committed to the dignity of BW should be seen as part of a broader project of social transformation – one that extends beyond institutional walls and is built through the collective construction of knowledge and political practice.

Reflective Activity

Having read the chapter, we invite you to reflect on your key learning and its implications for your professional practice as a nurse or midwife using Bain et al.'s (2002) 5R framework (p. 13–15):

- Reporting – What is it in your situation you want to transform after reading this chapter?
- Responding – What are your personal observations regarding your own situation/context in relation to what is raised in this chapter?
- Relating – What is/are the theoretical/research/data/legislative, etc., understandings relationship to under consideration in this chapter that you could apply to your situation/context?
- Reasoning – Identify how the chapter findings matter to your situation/context and how will you interrogate your situation/context and what will help you from this chapter?
- Reconstructing – Identify your action plans to reframe and rebuild a transformative way forward to change from the situation in your context.

References

Aguiar, C.D.A., Lopes, G.A., Bussadori, J.C.D.C., Leister, N., Riesco, M.L.G. and Alonso, B.D. (2025). Model of care in Brazilian out-of-hospital birth centers: A scoping review. Ciência & Saúde Coletiva, *30*, e09382023. https://doi.org/10.1590/1413-81232025301.09382023

Akotirene, C. (2018). *What is intersectionality?* Editora Jandaira.

American Anthropological Association. (2023). *Dr. Dána-Ain Davis*. https://americananthro.org/people/dr-dana-ain-davis/

Anunciação, D., Pereira, L.L., Silva, H.P., Nunes, A.P.N. and Soares, J.O. (2022). (Mis)paths in ensuring the health of the Black population and confronting racism in Brazil. Ciência & Saúde Coletiva, *27*, 3861–3870. https://doi.org/10.1590/1413-812320222710.08212022

Araújo, C.L.F., Campos, H.F. and Cardoso, M.M.V.N. (2019). *Social impact of the continuing education of obstetric nurses in Brazil: Experiences and innovative experiences after the professional qualification course – EEAN/UFRJ*. Rona Editora.

Bain, J.D., Ballantyne, R., Mills, C. and Lester, N.C. (2002). *Reflecting on practice: Students teachers' perspectives*. Post Pressed.

Bessa, R., Eleone, A., Freitas, R., Tavares, S. and Coelho, R. (2023). *Maternal mortality: causes and ways to cope*. https://ieps.org.br/wp-content/uploads/2023/03/olhar-IEPS-4-mortalidade-materna.pdf

Brazil, Instituto Brasileiro de Geografia e Estatística (IBGE). (2024). Portaria IBGE-1.041, de 28 de agosto de 2024. https://static.poder360.com.br/2024/08/dou-ibge-habitantes-brasil-29ago2024.pdf

Brazil, Ministry of Health. (1975). Programa Nacional de Imunizações (National Immunization Program). https://www.gov.br/saude/pt-br/acesso-a-informacao/acoes-e-programas/pni/pni

Brazil, Ministry of Health. (1990). Lei n° 8.080, de 19 de setembro de 1990. *Provides for the conditions necessary for the promotion, protection, and restoration of health*. https://www.planalto.gov.br/ccivil_03/leis/l8080.htm

Brazil, Ministry of Health. (1998). Lei n° 9.656, de 3 de junho de 1998. *Providers for private health care plans and insurance*. https://www.planalto.gov.br/ccivil_03/leis/l9656.htm

Brazil, Ministry of Health. (1999). Portaria n° 985/GM. https://www.saude.sp.gov.br/resources/humanizacao/biblioteca/leis/parto-e-nascimento/portaria_985_1999_cpn.pdf

Brazil, Ministry of Health. (2009). Guia de vigilância epidemiológica do óbito materno (Maternal death epidemiological surveillance guide). Ministério da Saúde.

Brazil, Ministry of Health. (2011a). Atenção ao pré-natal de baixo risco. Caderno de Atenção Básica (32 Low-risk prenatal care. Primary Care Notebook, 32). Ministério da Saúde.

Brazil, Ministry of Health. (2011b). Política Nacional de Atenção Integral à Saúde da Mulher: Princípios e diretrizes (National Policy for Comprehensive Women's Health Care: Principles and guidelines). Ministério da Saúde.

Brazil, Ministry of Health. (2014.) Atenção à saúde do recém-nascido: Guia para os profissionais de saúde (Newborn health care: A guide for health professionals). Ministério da Saúde.

Brazil, Ministry of Health. (2016). Política nacional de saúde integral da população negra: Uma política para o SUS (National comprehensive health policy for the Black population: A policy for the Unified Health System (SUS)). Ministério da Saúde.

Brazil, Ministry of Health. (2021). Maior sistema público de saúde do mundo, SUS completa 31 anos (The world's largest public health system, SUS, turns 31). https://www.gov.br/saude/pt-br/assuntos/noticias/2021/setembro/maior-sistema-publico-de-saude-do-mundo-sus-completa-31-anos

Brazil, Ministry of Health. (2022). Atenção primária e atenção especializada: Conheça os níveis de assistência do maior sistema público de saúde do mundo (Primary care and specialized care: Learn about the levels of care provided by the world's largest public health system). https://www.gov.br/saude/pt-br/assuntos/noticias/2022/marco/atencao-primaria-e-atencao-especializada-conheca-os-niveis-de-assistencia-do-maior-sistema-publico-de-saude-do-mundo

Brazil, Ministry of Health. (2023a). Manual de gestação de alto risco (High-Risk Pregnancy Manual). Ministério da Saúde.

Brazil, Ministry of Health. (2023b). Boletim epidemiológico sobre a saúde da população Negra (Epidemiological bulletin on the health of the Black population). Ministério da Saúde.

Brazil, Ministry of Health. (2023c) Relatório: Oficina de morte materna de mulheres negras no contexto do SUS (Report: Workshop on maternal deaths of Black women in the context of the Unified Health System (SUS)). Ministério da Saúde.

Brazil, Ministry of Health. (2024a). Portaria GM/MS n° 5.350, de 12 de setembro de 2024 (GM/MS Ordinance No. 5,350, of September 12, 2024). https://bvsms.saude.gov.br/bvs/saudelegis/gm/2024/prt5350_13_09_2024.html

Brazil, Ministry of Health. (2024b). Rede Alyne: Conheça a história da jovem negra que deu nome ao novo programa de cuidado integral à gestante e bebê (Alyne Network: Learn about the young Black woman who gave her name to the new comprehensive care program for pregnant women and babies). https://www.gov.br/saude/pt-br/assuntos/noticias/2024/setembro/rede-alyne-conheca-a-historia-da-jovem-negra-que-deu-nome-ao-novo-programa-de-cuidado-integral-a-gestante-e-bebe

Brazil, Ministry of Health. (2025). Relatório da Oficina Morte Materna das Mulheres Negras no Contexto do SUS (Report of the Workshop on Maternal Death of Black Women in the Context of the Unified Health System (SUS)). Ministério da Saúde.

Brazil, National Supplementary Health Agency (ANS). (2023). Indicadores da Dimensão Qualidade em Atenção à Saúde – IDQS. https://www.gov.br/ans/pt-br/assuntos/informacoes-e-avaliacoes-de-operadoras/indicadores-do-ano-base-2023

Carraca Pitta, B., de Sousa, I.C.F., Bez, F.F., Pertinhez, S.S., Lopes, G.P., Moreira, G.F., Carmona, V.S., Teixeira, U.H.G.F., Perin, L.C.B., Neves, T.N.A.B., Aguiar, J.M., Vitorino, K.L.C.L., dos Santos, F.C., Ribeiro, M.A.M. and Sattler, A.L. (2024). Transformations in childbirth care in Brazil: Challenges and perspectives for humanization with the participation of doulas and midwives. Periódicos Brasil Pesquisa Científica, *3*(2), 291–308. https://doi.org/10.36557/pbpc.v3i2.71

Carregal, F.A.S., Schreck, R.S.C., Santos, F.B.O. and Peres, M.A.A. (2020). Resgate histórico dos avanços da enfermagem obstétrica brasileira. História da Enfermagem Revista Eletrônica [Internet], *11*(2), 123–32. https://pesquisa.bvsalud.org/portal/resource/pt/biblio-1292061

Coelho, M., Mrejen, M., Remédios, J. and Campos, G. (2022). *Racial inequalities in health: Prenatal care and maternal mortality in Brazil, 2014–2020*. IEPS. https://ieps.org.br/nota-tecnica-27/

Costa, L.S., Rosa, S.Y.S., Souto, W.R. and Júnior, H.M.P.L. (2024). Nursing care focused on the maternal health of Black women. *Revista Ibero-Americana de Humanidades, Ciências e Educação, 10*, 1680–1694. https://doi.org/10.51891/rease.v10i4.13685

Crenshaw, K. (2002). Document for the meeting of experts on gender-related aspects of racial discrimination. Estudos Feministas Florianópolis, *10*(1), 171–188. https://www.scielo.br/j/ref/a/mbTpP4SFXPnJZ397j8fSBQQ/?format=pdf&lang=pt

Davis, D.A. (2018). The labor of racism. https://anthrodendum.org/2018/05/07/the-labor-of-racism/

Davis, D.A. (2019). Obstetric racism: The racial politics of pregnancy, labor, and birthing. *Medical Anthropology, 38*, 560–573. https://doi.org/10.1080/01459740.2018.1549389

Davis, D.A. (2020). Reproducing while Black: The crisis of Black maternal health, obstetric racism and assisted reproductive technology. *Reproductive Biomedicine & Society Online, 11*, 56–64. https://doi.org/10.1016/j.rbms.2020.10.001

Favelas News Agency. (2024). A booklet on obstetric violence and racism is created in Rio de Janeiro. ANF – Favelas News Agency. https://www.anf.org.br/cartilha-sobre-violencia-e-racismo-obstetrico-e-criada-no-rio-de-janeiro/

Fernandes, F. (1972). O negro no mundo dos brancos (The Black man in the White man's world). Difusão Européia do Livro.

Ferreira, T. (2023). Pequeno manual anti-rracismo obstétrico (Booklet on obstetric anti-racism). https://tribunadaimprensapopular.com.br/wp-content/uploads/2024/04/PEQUENO-MANUAL-DE-ANTI-RRACISMO-OBSTETRICO-1-1.pdf

Fiocruz. (2019). Principais questões sobre ambientes de atenção ao parto (Key issues regarding childbirth care environments). https://portaldeboaspraticas.iff.fiocruz.br/atencao-mulher/principais-questoes-sobre-ambientes-de-atencao-ao-parto/

Fiocruz. (2023). Violência obstétrica: Conceitos e evidências (Obstetric violence: Concepts and evidence). https://portaldeboaspraticas.iff.fiocruz.br/wp-content/uploads/2023/08/VIOLENCIA_OBSTETRICA.pdf

Fiocruz and COFEN. (2017). Perfil da enfermagem no Brasil: Relatório final da pesquisa. Vol. I – Brasil (Nursing profile in Brazil: Final research report. Vol. I – Brazil). Fiocruz/COFEN.

Goes, E.F. (2023). Dilemas interseccionais: Racismo e aborto no Brasil (Intersectional dilemmas: Racism and abortion in Brazil). Cadernos De Gênero E Diversidade, *9*(1), 31–46. https://doi.org/10.9771/cgd.v9i1.54896

Gonzalez, L. (2020). Por um feminismo afro-latino-americano. Zahar.

Higher Education Chamber of the National Council of Education. (2024). Revisão das Diretrizes Curriculares Nacionais para os cursos de graduação em enfermagem. https://coordenagraduacao.ufes.br/diretrizes-curriculares-nacionais

hooks, b. (1994). *Teaching to transgress* (Ensinando a transgredir). Routledge.

IBGE – Brazilian Institute of Geography and Statistics. (2022). Demographic Census 2022: Ethnic-racial identification of the population, by sex and age: Universe results. Ministry of Planning and Budget. https://biblioteca.ibge.gov.br/visualizacao/periodicos/3105/cd_2022_etnico_racial.pdf

Koga, G. (2022). Único no País, curso de Obstetrícia da USP reforça necessidade de parto seguro e humanizado (The only one in the country, the USP Obstetrics course reinforces the need for safe and humanized childbirth). *Jornal Da USP*. https://jornal.usp.br/universidade/unico-no-pais-curso-de-obstetricia-da-usp-reforca-necessidade-de-parto-seguro-e-humanizado/

Leal, M.C., Gama, S.G.N., Pereira, A.P.E., Pacheco, V.E., Carmo, C.N. and Santos, R.V. (2017). A cor da dor: Iniquidades raciais na atenção pré-natal e ao parto no Brasil (The color of pain: Racial inequities in prenatal and childbirth care in Brazil). *Cadernos de Saúde Pública, 33*(Suppl 1). https://doi.org/10.1590/0102-311X00078816

Leite, T.H., Marques, E.S., Esteves-Pereira, A.P., Nucci, M.F., Portella, Y. and Leal, M.C. (2022). Desrespeitos e abusos, maus tratos e violência obstétrica: Um desafio para a epidemiologia e a saúde pública no Brasil (Disrespect and abuse, mistreatment and obstetric violence: A challenge for epidemiology and public health in Brazil). *Ciência & Saúde Coletiva, 27*(2), 483–491. https://doi.org/10.1590/1413-81232022272.38592020

Lima, K.D.D., Pimentel, C. and Lyra, T.M. (2021). Disparidades raciais: Uma análise da violência obstétrica em mulheres negras (Racial disparities: An analysis of obstetric violence against Black women). *Ciência & Saúde Coletiva, 26*(Suppl 3), 4909–4918. https://doi.org/10.1590/1413-812320212611.3.24242019

National Health Council. (2017). Resolução n° 569. https://www.gov.br/conselho-nacional-de-saude/pt-br/acesso-a-informacao/atos-normativos/resolucoes/2017/resolucao-no-569.pdf

National Health Council. (2024). Rede Alyne: Novo programa busca reduzir mortalidade materna no Brasil (Alyne Network: New program seeks to reduce maternal mortality in Brazil). https://www.gov.br/conselho-nacional-de-saude/pt-br/assuntos/noticias/rede-alyne-novo-programa-busca-reduzir-mortalidade-materna-no-brasil

Paixão, M., Rossetto, I., Montovanele, F. and Carvano, L.M. (2010). Relatório anual das desigualdades raciais no Brasil 2009–2010: Constituição cidadã, seguridade social e seus efeitos sobre as assimetrias de cor ou raça (Annual report on racial inequalities in Brazil 2009–2010: Citizen constitution, social security and their effects on color or race asymmetries). https://dssbr.ensp.fiocruz.br/wp-content/uploads/2012/01/desigualdades_raciais_2009-2010.pdf

Palharini, L.A. and Figueirôa, S.F.M. (2018). Gênero, história e medicalização do parto: A exposição "Mulheres e práticas de saúde" (Gender, history and medicalization of childbirth: The exhibition "Women and Health Practices"). História, Ciências, Saúde – Manguinhos, *25*(4), 1039–1061. https://doi.org/10.1590/S0104-59702018000500008

Rebouças, P., Paixão, E.S., Ramos, D., Pescarini, J., Pinto-Junior, E.P., Falcão, I.R., Ichihara, M.Y., Sena, S., Veiga, R., Ribeiro, R., Rodrigues, L.C., Barreto, M.L. and Goes, E.F. (2024). Ethno-racial inequalities on adverse birth and neonatal outcomes: A nationwide, retrospective cohort study of 21 million Brazilian newborns. *Lancet Regional Health. Americas, 37*, 100833. https://doi.org/10.1016/j.lana.2024.100833

Ribeiro, D. (2017). O que é lugar de fala? (*What is a place of speech?*). Belo Horizonte.

Rodrigues, A.A. (2020). "É racismo que está aqui, e é isso que vai pautar até o fim": o ativismo de mulheres negras sobre violência obstétrica ("It's racism that's here, and that's what will guide us until the end": Black women's activism on obstetric violence). https://www.iff.fiocruz.br/index.php/pt/teses-e-dissertacoes?view=article&id=699:e-racismo-que-esta-aqui-e-e-isso-que-vai-pautar-ate-o-fim-o-ativismo-de-mulheres-negras-sobre-violencia-obstetrica&catid=37

Santos, I.O., Teixeira, E.C.C., Lopes, G.C., Silva, I.S. and Barbosa, S.V. (2024). Injustiças reprodutivas: Desigualdades no acesso a direitos sexuais e reprodutivos no Brasil. *Práticas e Cuidado: Revista De Saúde Coletiva, 5*, e20543. https://doi.org/10.5281/zenodo.13919713. https://revistas.uneb.br/index.php/saudecoletiva/article/view/20543

Silva, D.F.L., Lyra, T.M., Silva, J.B.R. and Faustino, D.M. (2023). Para além do racismo institucional? Uma análise do conteúdo da política de saúde para a população Negra (Beyond institutional racism? An analysis of the content of health policy for the Black population). *Ciência & Saúde Coletiva, 28*(9), 2527–2535. https://doi.org/10.1590/1413-81232023289.11602022

Souza, D.H., Rocha, D.G. and Nunes, N.R.A. (2024). Saúde da população negra na formação em saúde: Perspectivas rumo à equidade racial (Black population health in health education: Perspectives towards racial equity). *Ciência & Saúde Coletiva, 29*(7), e02992024. https://www.scielosp.org/article/csc/2024.v29n7/e02992024/

Souza, L.V. (2023). Parteiras, enfermeiras obstétricas e obstetrizes e a qualificação da atenção ao parto no Brasil desde o século XIX (Midwives, obstetric nurses and midwives and the qualification of childbirth care in Brazil since the 19th century). Fundo de População das Nações Unidas.

Tempesta, G.A. and Eneile, M. (2021). Racismo obstétrico: A política racial da gravidez, do parto e do Nascimento (Obstetric racism: The racial politics of pregnancy, labor, and birth). *Amazônica – Revista De Antropologia, 12*(2), 751. http://dx.doi.org/10.18542/amazonica.v12i2.9194

Werneck, J. (2016). Racismo institucional e saúde da população Negra (Institutional racism and the health of the Black population). Saúde e Sociedade, *25*(3), 535–549. https://doi.org/10.1590/S0104-129020162610

World Health Organization (WHO). (2015). *Declaração da OMS sobre taxas de cesáreas* (WHO statement on cesarean section rates). WHO.

Zanardo, G.L.P., Uribe, M.C., Nadal, A.H.R. and Habigzang, L.F. (2017). Violência obstétrica no Brasil: Uma revisão narrative (Obstetric violence in Brazil: A narrative review). *Psicologia & Sociedade, 29*, e155043. https://doi.org/10.1590/1807-0310/2017v29155043

9

CHANGING AUSTRALIAN NURSING AND MIDWIFERY

Undoing Decades of Racism in Healthcare

Tracy Reibel and Rhonda Marriott

Introduction

This chapter addresses challenges and responses to eliminating racism in Australian nursing and midwifery. Historically marginalised in healthcare access and healthcare professions, racism impacts First Peoples as patients and as health professionals. We highlight what has or is being changed, for example, in policy and professional practice, to promote anti-racism in health systems and professions. With higher preterm and low birthweight infant outcomes, from birth Aboriginal and Torres Strait Islander peoples[1] experience significant life course health inequities. Encountering racism when seeking healthcare is well documented; leading to, for example, discharge against medical advice and disengagement from mainstream health services.

While there is evidence of stated commitments to dismantling institutional racism in the Australian health system and professions, there is also evidence of its ongoing presence. For the system to address health inequities experienced by First Peoples, the elimination of racism is a crucial element of change, alongside increased numbers of First Peoples health professionals. Additionally, concerted efforts are required to rethink health professional education and practice and prioritise cultural safety[2] in all education and health settings.

Background

In 2004 Henry et al. (p. 517), quoted McConnachie et al. (1988) definition of institutional racism as, "the ways in which racist beliefs or values have been built into the operations of social institutions in such a way as to discriminate against, control and oppress various minority groups", adding racism may be covert or

DOI: 10.4324/9781003565369-9

unrecognised. Providing examples of how racism is expressed in Australian healthcare, they noted funding inequities, different "performance" criteria being applied to Black and white healthcare organisations, inequitable Medicare[3] primary healthcare and cultural barriers to First Peoples' use of mainstream healthcare services. In the 20 years since, strategies and actions are evident across government, regulators and professional bodies.

First Peoples' *self-determined change* began with the first Aboriginal medical service established in Redfern, New South Wales in 1971. Since then, the Aboriginal Community Controlled Health Organisations (ACCHOs) sector has grown to over 146 health services in metropolitan and regional locations in all states and territories, many with multiple clinics covering broad areas of health service delivery to address unmet need. The sector provides primary care and support and referral services to specialists. Despite this profoundly important initiative, in 2025, 270 years since the British crown took possession of "Australia", change is slow. ACCHOs continue to manage cultural barriers to healthcare while ensuring availability of culturally safe care, especially for underserved communities in rural, remote and very remote locations despite funding inequities. Further, according to the Australian Institute of Health and Welfare (AIHW), with lower access to health services than non-Indigenous Australians, differential outcomes between non-Indigenous and First Peoples' life expectancy persist; 8.8 years for males and 8.1 years for females, with males and females living in remote and very remote areas having the lowest life expectancy, while the highest was in inner and outer regional areas, followed closely by major cities (AIHW 2025).

A key solution to redressing health inequities is challenging institutional racism in mainstream primary, secondary and tertiary health services – still considered complex with meaningful change difficult to implement. This is partially due to Australia's split legislative responsibilities, with the federal government responsible for delivery of general practice primary healthcare, including via ACCHOs, and state/territory governments responsible for hospital services and specialist care delivery, leading to fragmented care.

In this chapter, we focus on racism in Australia's health system and professions requiring long-term strategic and coordinated commitments by governments, professional bodies and individual professionals taking responsibility for the inequities experienced by First Peoples; and working collaboratively with First Peoples' advisory bodies to make change.

How health systems frame and deliver care and the mechanisms used to achieve health equity rely on eliminating institutional racism. Institutions can and should set clear workforce strategies, including establishing acceptable professional behaviour and what will not be tolerated, with appropriate measures in place when failure to provide non-judgemental, equitable and high-quality care is identified. Individual professionals must take responsibility for ensuring their practice does not discriminate based on race, gender or religion. Each needs to be aware, or be made aware, of the impact of their conscious/unconscious bias towards other cultures, how it is evident in their practice and how it impacts patients in their care. Without this personal responsibility, health system change will remain unrealised.

This chapter highlights the significant advocacy undertaken by Aboriginal and Torres Strait Islander peoples and organisations, instrumental in strategies being implemented by governments and professional bodies to directly address the harm caused by racism.

Call to Action (the Call) For Anti-Racism Change

Responding to the global Black Lives Matter (BLM) movement, in 2020 over 100 Aboriginal and Torres Strait Islander and non-Indigenous nursing and midwifery leaders were signatories to *A Unified Call to Action from Australian Nursing and Midwifery Leaders: Ensuring that Black Lives Matter* (Geia et al. 2020). The introduction references the death of Mr. George Floyd in the USA, with protests across Australia using the slogans "Black Lives Matter" and "I can't breathe"; linking his death to the plight of incarcerated Aboriginal and Torres Strait Islander peoples, laid bare in the seminal Australian Royal Commission into Aboriginal Deaths in Custody 1998 (Commonwealth of Australia 2002).

That Royal Commission examined in depth the long history of Black deaths in custody; noting that First Peoples remain significantly over-represented in legal and correctional systems. The outcomes highlight how settler colonisers from the outset incarcerated First Peoples, denied their human rights, and until the 1967 federal government referendum to acknowledge First Peoples as equal citizens of Australia was passed, failed to understand First Peoples' 60,000 years plus of custodianship. Aboriginal people were pivotal in the 1967 referendum result, campaigning for 10 years prior, including one of the Call authors and signatories, Aunty Dulcie Flower AM. First Peoples' activists have a long and proud history of seeking change also evident in the 2024 Voice Referendum vote which, although lost, demonstrated that tireless advocacy continues to highlight dispossession of lands, culture, language and autonomy.

The Call goes on to discuss how the Royal Commission reporting of Aboriginal deaths in custody continues to be present in discussions of institutional racism. The signatories link the domination of whiteness to power imbalances against Black people with white privilege driving health disparities and an absence of cultural safety leading to health inequities. They note nursing and midwifery professions as complicit in continued racialised discourses and practices, requiring interrogation of the professions' history and frameworks of healthcare provision and the need to conduct difficult conversations about the founding philosophies, policies and practices impacting healthcare for First Peoples. Explicitly, the Call notes the coronial inquiry into the 2014 death in custody of Yamatji woman Miss Dhu in Western Australia, citing the institutionally racist standard of nursing care in the chain of events leading to her death; confirmed in the Coroner's inquest into her death, which found neglect and mistreatment by both police and hospital staff caused her "catastrophic decline".

Health Systems Efforts to Address Racism

Examples of health professions and government efforts to address racism in healthcare are reflected in various position statements. One example is a 2018 joint statement – *Cultural Safety: Nurses and Midwives Leading the Way for Safer Healthcare* – prepared by the Congress of Aboriginal and Torres Strait Islander Nurses and Midwives (CATSINaM), the Australian Nursing and Midwifery Board (ANMB), Australian College of Midwives (ACM), Australian College of Nursing (ACN) and Australian Nursing and Midwifery Federation (ANMF) that noted all leaders and health professionals working in healthcare have a role to play in closing the gap (Ahpra and the National Boards 2024, Commonwealth of Australia n.d.). The statement calls on the healthcare systems largest workforce to commit to codes of conduct, with individuals providing culturally safe, respectful care and practising open, honest and compassionate professional relationships (Milligan et al 2021). Another is the Office of the National Rural Health Commissioner Annual Report 2022–23. 2022-23 (Australian Government Office of the National Rural Health Commissioner 2023) in its statement acknowledging the impacts of racism on Indigenous Australians and its commitment to change. This includes: (i) working closely with Indigenous leaders and peak organisations to advise governments, medical institutions, colleges and universities to ensure racism is acknowledged and addressed; (ii) recommending governments, medical institutions, colleges and universities dismantle systemic barriers for Indigenous medical, nursing and allied health students to access, pursue and maintain a career in Australia's health system; and (iii) promoting cultural safety and responsiveness and the eradication of racism in the health sector experienced by consumers and workforce.

Selected from many examples, these statements demonstrate commitments to culturally safe care are a shared cross-sectorial goal. Nonetheless, the Australian health system continues to grapple with ongoing racism experienced by First Peoples, directly impacting their physical and mental health, referred to as social and emotional wellbeing (SEWB), a descriptor of the unique way in which Aboriginal and Torres Strait Islander peoples frame their health. According to Gee et al (2014), SEWB is a "multidimensional concept of health that includes mental health, but which also encompasses domains of health and wellbeing such as connection to land or 'country', culture, spirituality, ancestry, family, and community" (p. 55). In response to the ongoing advocacy of First Peoples' leaders, the process of reckoning to drive health systems and health professionals reform is ongoing.

Understanding the impacts of racism on First Peoples' health outcomes is one thing; how health systems and individual health professionals contribute to the elimination of racism is another. The Australian Health Practitioner Regulation Agency (Ahpra) and the National Boards (n.d.a) has an *Aboriginal and Torres*

Strait Islander Anti-Racism Policy providing detailed guidance relevant to understanding and addressing racism in everyday settings. Ahpra has a significant role to play in regulating practice to ensure Aboriginal and Torres Strait Islander peoples are treated equally (clinically and as individuals) in healthcare settings. The racism policy sits alongside Ahpra and the National Boards's (n.d. b & c, respectively) *Aboriginal and Torres Strait Islander Employment Strategy 2020–2025* and the *National Scheme's Aboriginal and Torres Strait Islander Health and Cultural Safety Strategy 2020–2025*.

What though do statements or strategies have on First Peoples' health outcomes or their participation in the workforce? As noted by Thackrah et al (2021) and Topp et al (2022), the persistence of racism in healthcare is an unresolved issue, requiring responses in the professions and in health systems to combat racism. While there is resistance to change or an inability of non-Indigenous health professionals to acknowledge biases in their perceptions of First Peoples, effective care will not be available (Laccos-Barrett et al 2022).

What follows is an evidence synthesis interrogating actions Australian nursing and midwifery professions are formulating to address racism; including educating new generations of culturally safe healthcare professionals as agents of change in making health systems better for First Peoples. Rix et al (2024) also refer to the need for white nurse educators to unlearn what they know about First Peoples and their health needs, decolonising their perspectives and finding new approaches in professional practice (Kotz et al. 2025).

Drivers of Anti-Racism Change

Closing the Gap

The negative impact of racism on First People's life course health goes back decades, underpinning the long-time advocacy of peak bodies including CATSINaM and the National Aboriginal Community Controlled Health Organisation (NACCHO). NACCHO noted in 2020, as determined through the Australian Reconciliation Barometer – a national study by Reconciliation Australia conducted every two years – the global and local BLM movements challenged the experiences and understanding of racism in Australia, with the broader Australian society's understanding of racism heightened. Consequently, NACCHO developed a National Anti-Racism Framework, submitted to the Australian Human Rights Commission in February 2022. Six recommendations included an alignment of the Anti-Racism Framework with the National Agreement on Closing the Gap (NACtG), recognition of the impact of racism on the health and wellbeing of Aboriginal and Torres Strait Islander peoples and accreditation standards used to embed cultural safety in healthcare services (Government of Western Australia 2015, National Aboriginal Community Controlled Health Organisation 2022).

The first Federal Government Closing the Gap statement in 1990 led to the 2020 NACtG – agreed by a coalition of First Peoples peak bodies, all state premiers/territory chief ministers and the Australian Local Government Association – against which governments would report annually (Australian Government 2020, 2025). The NaCtG explicitly sets out the conditions for achieving social and health equity for Aboriginal and Torres Strait Islander peoples. Together with four Priority Reforms (1) formal partnerships and shared decision making; (2) building the community-controlled sector; (3) transforming government organisation; and (4) shared access to data and information at the regional level, 17 socio-economic outcome areas were cross referenced to the Priority Reforms. Each outcome has associated targets, indicators/drivers, disaggregation guidance and data development. While the outcomes emphasise health, education and justice, many of the individual outcomes concern the social determinants and delivery of health. Recent NACtG reporting demonstrates little improvement in First Nations outcomes (Uniting NSW.ACT 2025).

Nursing and Midwifery Workforce

Australian government (2022) acknowledged some time ago that health equity is dependent on growing the Aboriginal and Torres Strait Islander health workforce. According to West et al (2016) the Indigenous Nursing Education Working Group (INEWG) in 2002 had called for a national strategic approach to increase the number of graduates from mainstream nursing programs. The authors noted that "program completion rates have not kept pace with increased enrolments and remain lower for Aboriginal and Torres Strait Islander nursing students compared to other Australian students" (p. 349–10). They noted the primary reasons for this outcome: financial hardship, *institutional racism* and academics who lack awareness and understanding of students' cultural obligations. Even so, their assessment of available data at the time showed significant improvements in Indigenous nursing student completions between 2002 and 2014, suggesting focussed strategies achieve outcomes.

By 2021 Coleman et al., noted an under representation of Aboriginal people entering midwifery education and the workforce. From a workforce perspective, in 2015 Aboriginal midwives were 1% (n=189) of the midwifery workforce across Australia with CATSINaM at that time having a stated aim of achieving midwifery workforce parity (n=600+). The 2023/24 Aphra Nursing and Midwifery Board report notes 1.6% (or 552) of the total midwifery workforce (34,510) identified as Aboriginal and/or Torres Strait Islander. While this number does not meet the CATSINaM goal, a positive trend is evident. However, this relatively small number of midwives is spread across seven states and territories, leaving many maternity services across the nation without any Aboriginal and Torres Strait Islander midwives. AIHW reported in 2021 that First Peoples represented 3.8% of the total population and in 2023 were 8.6% of all births. It is well established that women require good antenatal care to achieve a healthy birthweight infant and avoid premature or still births. Aboriginal and Torres Strait Islander women remain overrepresented in adverse perinatal outcomes; underlining the necessity of growing the Aboriginal and Torres Strait Islander midwifery workforce to support perinatal women to feel confident and safe to access care. Coleman et al (2021) reference access to culturally safe maternity care through cultural safety practiced by non-Indigenous midwives as another crucial strategic approach to promoting service engagement by First Peoples' women.

For First Peoples' undertaking health professional careers, most, if not all, Aboriginal and Torres Strait Islander people who decide on a nursing and midwifery career are motivated by their desire to "support mob"[4]; reflected in Springall et al's qualitative study (2025) which considered the impact of current strategies to improve recruitment and retention of First Peoples midwifery students. Their study notes students prefer mentorships with fellow nursing or midwifery mob to assist them to feel culturally safe and protected. Also noted was a desire to create a birth space for First Peoples families in their care facilitated by their capacity to immediately connect with their patients because they understand how families feel when they go into a hospital. Of high relevance was that students described how racism, white privilege and oppression impacts them and their studies; requiring them to "adapt their thinking" (also referred to as code switching) to address the challenge of working in institutions which are "systematically racist". It is evident that student motivation is quickly sapped by education and health systems that students, and graduates, are required to work within to achieve their aims of supporting mob. These and other factors contribute to poor retention of graduates in mainstream health systems, in turn impacting the healthcare that First Peoples' families receive.

Retention of Nurses and Midwives

Many strategies have been proposed to enhance retention of nursing and midwifery students. While First People enrolments and graduations in nursing and midwifery are incrementally increasing, retaining graduates in the health workforce is problematic. Lai et al (2018) in their review of factors affecting the retention of First Peoples in the health workforce concluded that building a strong health workforce requires not only recruitment into health careers but what happens after recruitment is equally important for the health system to retain that workforce. This includes culturally safe workplaces, encompassing the attitudes of health leaders and coworkers, with access to supervision, mentoring and training. Another review by Taylor et al (2019) focused on retention of Aboriginal and Torres Strait Islander health students, articulating a suite of measures needed to provide support, such as pre-entry preparation programs, and cultural support and strong organisational leadership available across the undergraduate years, to enable students to overcome any challenges impacting their educational participation and ensure they graduate as health professionals.

A focus on health education and health system environments in which First Peoples' feel culturally safe and supported is essential to increasing workforce retention. While the studies cited above consider the impact of mentoring programs, curriculum changes which facilitate culturally safe teaching and learning for Aboriginal and Torres Strait Islander peoples are also needed. For example, Murdoch University in Western Australia (WA) is currently developing a *School of Nursing Strategy for First Nations Students (Undergraduate, Postgraduate and Research)*. Drawing on the core principles of the *Aboriginal and Torres Strait Islander Health Curriculum Framework* (AdoHaAC (Australian Government, 2014; CATSINaM 2017) and the *WA Aboriginal Health and Wellbeing Framework* (WAAHWF (Government of Western Australia, 2015)). The stated aim of this educational innovation is to create entry pathways to nursing courses as the university of choice for Aboriginal people in WA. Premised on a new philosophical approach to strengths-based teaching and learning, the new curriculum structure is a deliberate move away from the biomedical/deficit approach currently dominating nursing and midwifery curricula.

Biles et al noted in a 2023 scoping review that culturally safe mentoring has been a key recommendation in the nursing literature for over 20 years, albeit with limited knowledge of what constitutes an effective program. A previous qualitative study (2021) with Aboriginal nurses and midwives in one local health district in New South Wales (NSW) – Australia's most populous state – focused on perceptions of mentors and mentees, including the barriers and enablers to participating in such a program. From this, Biles et al described foundational insights for effective mentoring programs. These include participants feeling safe and empowered to speak out against racism. They linked this outcome to a NSW Health employee survey noting ~25% of employees experienced racism in the workplace from a colleague. From the learnings of this study, an extended mentoring program – Deadly Aboriginal and Torres Strait Islander Nursing and Midwifery Mentoring (DANMN) program (Biles et al 2024) was established. Available across five diverse NSW health districts, the DANMN project aligns with local and statewide health plans and strategies, addressing the critical issues of workforce cultural safety and retention. Premised on Aboriginal ways of knowing, being and doing, the approach seeks to acknowledge the historical, present and ongoing impact of Western colonisation on Aboriginal peoples, cultures and lands.

Aboriginal and Torres Strait Islander Nurses and Midwives Experiences of Racism

The lived experience of Aboriginal and Torres Strait Islander students and graduates in nursing and midwifery is reflected in three recent studies. One focussed on nurses and the other two on midwives and all demonstrate the ongoing need for change in health systems, to make these culturally safe spaces for Aboriginal and Torres Strait Islander nurses and midwives to work within.

Best et al (2025) investigated the detrimental effects of racism on Aboriginal and Torres Strait Islander nurses' professional trajectories, sense of self within the healthcare environment and overall well-being. In their assessment, few studies have considered the perspectives of First Peoples nurses and that racism in the workplace is rarely researched, interrogated or challenged. Further, racism in health is a significant challenge to recruitment and retention and needs to be examined and understood. Best et al's qualitative study suggested a correlation between nurses' length of experience and their willingness to confront racist incidents, while also highlighting the deleterious impacts that acting against racism can have on individuals. They conclude that racism harms Aboriginal and Torres Strait Islander nurses' careers, identity, safety and social and emotional well-being; and that bearing the consequences of working in a culturally unsafe health system is exhausting. The authors propose a new concept in the term **racism fatigue** which encapsulates nurses experience of this persistent and emotionally draining problem which ultimately leads them to leave their profession. The concept sits alongside the **cultural load** (Sivertsen et al 2023) experienced by First Peoples' nurses and midwives who, despite their small numbers in individual health services, are frequently expected to assume the role of cultural contact for all First Peoples' patients attending a service, thereby increasing their work burden.

Hartz et al (2025) scoping review on the experiences of Aboriginal and Torres Strait Islander midwifery students and midwives identified four peer reviewed qualitative research papers, confirming Best et al's (2025) summation of too few studies on this important topic. Hartz and colleagues expanded their search to include grey literature from reputable sources that met their criteria. Three interconnected themes emerged: connection and kinship, racism and balancing responsibilities, concluding these aspects as foundational in providing experiences for Aboriginal and Torres Strait Islander midwives and midwifery students that are clinically and academically transformational, culturally safe and promote resilience. The theme of connection refers to the capacity for midwives and students to connect with each other and how they value working with their peers; while the theme of racism refers to the need for culturally safe clinical, work and study environments which both respect Aboriginal and Torres Strait Islander midwives and students and actively oppose racism in the personal, community and organisational interfaces (Taylor et al. 2020). In an earlier integrative literature review, Coleman et al., (2021) had identified only three articles available at the time relevant to assessing the experiences of First Peoples' midwifery students. The authors expanded their search to include Aboriginal undergraduate health students, which increased the number of relevant papers to nine, and incorporated papers focussed on nursing, psychology and medical students; identifying key themes as cultural safety, kinship and support. Hartz and colleagues subsequent 2025 scoping review focussed solely on midwives and midwifery students. The authors noted the following components as crucial to cultural safety education reformation aimed at creating better conditions for

First People's participation in nursing and midwifery education. These include connections (as promoted by mentorship, Aboriginal peer academics, clinical training in ACCHOs), flexible learning modules, including online and placements close to home locations, targeted clinical placements in First Peoples' models of care and cadetships and scholarships, noted as available in four of six states and two territories.

The education of the next generation of nurses and midwives is therefore dependent on educators developing and delivering curricula which reflect the needs of Aboriginal and Torres Strait Islander students. As noted earlier, innovations in this space are emerging. However, there is no available evidence at the time of writing to demonstrate this is widespread across the Australian university nursing and midwifery education sector.

Cultural Safety Is the Change Needed to Eliminate Racism in Healthcare

In 2018 the Nursing and Midwifery Board declared that cultural safety and dignified care should be the guiding cornerstones for nurses and midwives work. This was required to better serve and mirror the cultures of the Aboriginal and Torres Strait Islander peoples; to deliver authentic service provision and improved collaborative and partnership working between health and communities. Studies by Fleming et al (2017, 2019, 2020) reflect on midwifery academics' awareness of cultural safety, awareness of cultural safety in the midwifery workforce and cultural safety professional development for midwives. For example, their study with midwifery academics (2017) used a pre-post method to establish any shifts in understanding of cultural safety after exposure in two workshops (the intervention). The post intervention responses to the Awareness of Cultural Safety Scale score were significantly higher, while perceptions of racism showed no statistically significant differences pre and post.

These and other studies reflect our research with 71 midwives and midwifery educators in Western Australia which found that to achieve a culturally safe non-Indigenous workforce, workforce and health systems issues need to support individual midwives' capability to provide culturally safe care to Aboriginal women. Further, effective cultural education and improved professional accountability alongside significant changes in health systems, including culturally safe woman-centred care models, are key to addressing racism in healthcare (Marriott et al 2020; Marriott et al 2021).

Fleming et al (2019) followed up with an evaluation of awareness of cultural safety in the midwifery workforce using an adapted Awareness of Cultural Safety Scale – with measures including the revised scale, self-assessment of cultural knowledge and perceptions of racism scales. The authors concluded the revised scale was a reliable and valid measure of cultural safety across a diverse sample of midwives (n=92) and midwives working in education settings demonstrated a higher awareness of cultural safety than clinical peers. Fleming et al's final study (2020) examined the influence of yarning circles within a professional development program to enhance midwifery academics' awareness of cultural safety, find the yarning circles provided a safe and supportive space for challenging discussions.

Conclusion

As highlighted in this chapter, racism impacts First Peoples as patients and as health professionals. To redress this, long-term strategic and coordinated commitment is required by governments, professional bodies and individual professionals working collaboratively with First Peoples' advisory bodies to make change aligned with the NaCtG's four Priority Reforms together with commitments to grow and adequately fund the ACCHOs sector as preferred health service providers for First Peoples.

Aboriginal-led change in all education and health settings to prioritise cultural safety is essential. Building and retaining the Aboriginal and Torres Strait Islander health workforce and culturally safe environments will reduce racism fatigue and cultural load. Effective cultural education and improved professional accountability alongside significant changes in health systems to meet the needs of First Peoples healthcare are key to addressing racism.

Reflective Activity

Having read the chapter, we invite you to reflect on your key learning and its implications for your professional practice as a nurse or midwife using Bain et al.'s (2002) 5R framework (p. 13–15):

- Reporting – what is it in your situation you want to transform after reading this chapter?
- Responding – what are your personal observations regarding your own situation/context in relation to what is raised in this chapter?
- Relating – what is/are the theoretical/research/data/legislative, etc. understandings relationship to under consideration in this chapter that you could apply to your situation/context?
- Reasoning – identify how the chapter findings matter to your situation/context and how will you interrogate your situation/context and what will help you from this chapter.
- Reconstructing – identify your action plans to reframe and rebuild a transformative way forward to change from the situation in your context.

Notes

1 Aboriginal and Torres Strait Islander peoples are the First Peoples of Australia. In this chapter, we will use these terms interchangeably, Aboriginal in some contexts, and Indigenous/non-Indigenous when referring to or quoting from cited documents used in relation to Aboriginal and Torres Strait Islander peoples or non-Indigenous Australians.

2 Cultural safety is central to creating safe health care environments for Aboriginal and Torres Strait Islander peoples in the health system. Cultural safety describes a circumstance where people are enabled and feel they can access health care that suits their

needs, are able to challenge personal or institutional racism (when they experience it), establishes trust in services, and underpins effective, quality care – Indigenous Allied Health Australia) Policy Position Statement. https://iaha.com.au/wp-content/uploads/2020/02/Cultural-Safety-Through-Responsive-Health-Practice-Position-Statement.pdf accessed August 2025.

3 Medicare has been Australia's universal health care scheme since 1984 providing medical services, public hospitals and medicines https://www.health.gov.au/about-us/the-australian-health-system.

4 "Mob" is a term used by Aboriginal people to refer to Aboriginal and Torres Strait Islander peoples collectively and/or to a person's language group.

References

Australian Government. (2014). Aboriginal and Torres Strait Islander Health Curriculum Framework. Australian Government Department of Health, Disability and Ageing https://www.health.gov.au/sites/default/files/documents/2020/12/aboriginal-and-torres-strait-islander-health-curriculum-framework.pdf

Australian Government. (2022). *Position Statement: Impacts of racism on the health and wellbeing of Indigenous Australians*. Office of the National Rural Health Commissioner. https://www.health.gov.au/sites/default/files/documents/2022/03/position-statement-impacts-of-racism-on-the-health-and-wellbeing-of-indigenous-australians-impacts-of-racism-on-the-health-and-wellbeing-of-indigenous-australians.pdf.

Australian Government. (2020). *National Agreement on Closing the Gap July 2020*. Department of Prime Minister and Cabinet. https://www.closingthegap.gov.au/national-agreement/national-agreement-closing-the-gap

Australian Government Office of the National Rural Health Commissioner (2023). Office of the National Rural Health Commissioner Annual Report 2022–23. https://www.health.gov.au/resources/publications/annual-report-2022-23-office-of-the-national-rural-health-commissioner?language=en

Australian Government. (2025). Closing the Gap Commonwealth 2024 Annual Report Commonwealth 2025 Implementation Plan. https://www.niaa.gov.au/sites/default/files/documents/2025-02/NIAA%20CTG%20Combined%20Report.pdf

Australian Health Practitioner Regulation Agency (Ahpra) and the National Boards. (2024). *ANNUAL REPORT 2023/24 Leadership and collaboration for safer healthcare*. https://www.ahpra.gov.au/Publications/Annual-reports/Annual-report-2024.aspx

Australian Health Practitioner Regulation Agency (Ahpra) and the National Boards (n.d.a). *Aboriginal and Torres Strait Islander Anti-Racism Policy*.

Australian Health Practitioner Regulation Agency (Ahpra) and the National Boards (n.d.b). *Aboriginal and Torres Strait Islander Employment Strategy 2020–2025*.

Australian Health Practitioner Regulation Agency (Ahpra) and the National Boards (n.d.c). *National Scheme's Aboriginal and Torres Strait Islander Health and Cultural Safety Strategy 2020–2025*.

Australian Institute of Health and Welfare (AIHW). (2021). *Australia's welfare 2021: in brief. Cat. No. AUS 237*. AIHW. https://www.aihw.gov.au/getmedia/b5c49e10-c8c7-4629-b183-83354894204b/aihw-aus-237.pdf?v=20230605163346&inline=true

Australian Institute of Health and Welfare (AIHW). (2025). *Aboriginal and Torres Strait Islander Health Performance Framework - Summary report June 2025*. AIHW: Australian Government. https://www.indigenoushpf.gov.au/

Bain, J.D., Ballantyne, R., Mills, C. and Lester, N.C. (2002). *Reflecting on practice: Students teachers' perspectives*. Post Pressed.

Best, O., Bayliss, L., Hodgman, S. and Peters, M.D. (2025). Aboriginal and Torres Strait Islander nurses' experiences of racism at work. *Collegian, 32*(2), 61–68. doi: https://doi.org/10.1016/j.colegn.2024.12.004

Biles, J., Deravin, L., McMillan Am, F., Anderson, J., Sara, G. and Biles, B. (2023). Aboriginal and Torres Strait Islander nurses and midwives culturally safe mentoring programmes in Australia: A scoping review. *Contemporary Nurse*, *59*(2), 173–183. doi: https://doi.org/10.1080/10376178.2023.2175700.

Biles, B., Christian, B., Marshall, C., McMillan, F., Sara, G., Anderson, J., Davies, N., Fealy, S. and Biles, J. (2024). 'DANMM that's good!': evaluating the feasibility and acceptability of the Deadly Aboriginal and Torres Strait Islander Nursing and Midwifery Mentoring (DANMM) Programme across rural, regional and metropolitan NSW–a collaborative study protocol. *BMJ open*, *14*(2), p.e079416. doi: https://doi.org/10.1136/bmjopen-2023-079416

Congress of Aboriginal and Torres Strait Islander Nurses and Midwives (CATSINaM). (2017). *Nursing and Midwifery Aboriginal and Torres Strait Islander Health Curriculum Framework.* https://issuu.com/catsinam1/docs/nursing-and-midwifery-health-curriculum-framework_

Coleman, R., Hartz, D. and Dahlen, H. (2021). The experiences of Aboriginal and Torres Strait Islander Bachelor of Midwifery students: An integrative literature review. *Women and Birth*, *34*(1), 69–76. doi: https://doi.org/10.1016/j.nepr.2025.104409

Commonwealth of Australia. (2002). *Aboriginal deaths in custody: The Royal Commission and its records, 1987–91*. National Archives of Australia https://www.naa.gov.au/sites/default/files/2020-06/research-guide-aboriginal-deaths-in-custody_0.pdf

Commonwealth of Australia. (n.d.). *Commonwealth Closing the Gap Implementation Plan 2025* https://www.niaa.gov.au/resource-centre/commonwealth-closing-gap-2024-annual-report-and-2025-implementation-plan

Coroner's Court of Western Australia (2016). *Inquest Findings 2016 – Inquest into the Death of Ms DHU, 16 December 2016.* https://www.coronerscourt.wa.gov.au/I/inquest_into_the_death_of_ms_dhu.aspx?uid=6192-80-9559-3939

Fleming, T., Creedy, D.K. and West, R. (2017). Impact of a continuing professional development intervention on midwifery academics' awareness of cultural safety. *Women and Birth*, *30*(3), 245–252. doi: https://doi.org/10.1016/j.wombi.2017.02.004

Fleming, T., Creedy, D.K. and West, R. (2019). Cultural safety continuing professional development for midwifery academics: An integrative literature review. *Women and Birth*, *32*(4), 318–326. doi: https://doi.org/10.1016/j.wombi.2018.11.001

Fleming, T., Creedy, D.K. and West, R. (2020). The influence of yarning circles: A cultural safety professional development program for midwives. *Women and Birth*, *33*(2), 175–185. doi: https://doi.org/10.1016/j.wombi.2019.03.016

Gee, G., Dudgeon, P., Schultz, C., Hart, A. and Kelly, K. (2014). Aboriginal and Torres Strait Islander social and emotional wellbeing. In Dudgeon, P., Milroy, H., & Walker, R. *(editors) Working together: Aboriginal and Torres Strait Islander mental health and wellbeing principles and practice.* Australian Government Department of the Prime Minister and Cabinet (pp. 55–68). https://www.thekids.org.au/globalassets/media/documents/aboriginal-health/working-together-second-edition/wt-part-1-chapt-4-final.pdf

Geia, L., Baird, K., Bail, K., Barclay, L., Bennett, J., Best, O., Birks, M., Blackley, L., Blackman, R., Bonner, A., Bryant Ao, R., Buzzacott, C., Campbell, S., Catling, C., Chamberlain, C., Cox, L., Cross, W., Cruickshank, M., Cummins, A., Dahlen, H., … Wynne, R. (2020). A unified call to action from Australian nursing and midwifery leaders: ensuring that Black lives matter. *Contemporary nurse*, *56*(4), 297–308. https://doi.org/10.1080/10376178.2020.1809107

Government of Western Australia. (2015). *WA Aboriginal Health and Wellbeing Framework 2015–2030.* https://www.health.wa.gov.au/~/media/Files/Corporate/general-documents/Aboriginal-health/PDF/12853_WA_Aboriginal_Health_and_Wellbeing_Framework.pdf

Hartz, D.L., Coleman, R., Butcher, S., McGrath, L., Buzzacott, C., Williams, K., Coe, A. and Kosiak, M. (2025). What are the experiences of Aboriginal and/or Torres Strait Islander midwifery students and midwives? A scoping review. *Women and Birth, 38*(1), 101856. doi: https://doi.org/10.1016/j.wombi.2024.101856

Henry, B.R., Houston, S. and Mooney, G.H. (2004). Institutional racism in Australian healthcare: a plea for decency. *Medical Journal of Australia, 180*(10), 517–520. doi: 10.5694/j.1326-5377.2004.tb06056.x

Kotz, J., Reid, C., Robinson, M., Walker, R., Reibel, T., Bairnsfather-Scott, A. and Marriott, R. (2025). Decolonizing the exploration of perinatal mental health screening with Indigenous Australian parents in primary care. *Primary health care research & development, 26*, e66.

Laccos-Barrett, K., Brown, A.E., Saunders, V., Baldock, K.L. and West, R. (2022). Are we teaching nurses to be racist towards Aboriginal and Torres Strait Islander peoples? A critical race document analysis of discrete Aboriginal and Torres Strait Islander health courses. *International Journal of Environmental Research and Public Health, 19*(18), 11455. doi: https://doi.org/10.3390/ijerph191811455

Lai, G.C., Taylor, E.V., Haigh, M.M. and Thompson, S.C. (2018). Factors affecting the retention of indigenous Australians in the health workforce: a systematic review. *International journal of environmental research and public health, 15*(5), 914. doi: https://doi.org/10.3390/ijerph15050914

Marriott, R., Reibel, T., Gliddon, J., Griffin, D., Coffin, J., Eades, A.M., Robinson, M., Bowen, A., Kendall, S., Martin, T. and Monterosso, L. (2020). Aboriginal research methods and researcher reflections on working two-ways to investigate culturally secure birthing for Aboriginal women. *Australian Aboriginal Studies*, (1), 36–53.

Marriott, R., Reibel, T., Barrett, T.L., Bowen, A., Bradshaw, S., Kendall, S., Kotz, J., Martin, T., Monterosso, L. and Robinson, M. (2021). Midwifery knowledge of equitable and culturally safe maternity care for Aboriginal women. *Birth, 48*(1), pp. 132–138. https://doi.org/10.1111/birt.12525

McConnochie, K.R., Hollinsworth, D. and Pettman J. (1988). *Race & Racism in Australia.* Social Science Press.

Milligan, E., West, R., Saunders, V., Bialocerkowski, A., Creedy, D., Minniss, F.R., Hall, K. and Vervoort, S. (2021). Achieving cultural safety for Australia's First Peoples: a review of the Australian Health Practitioner Regulation Agency-registered health practitioners' Codes of Conduct and Codes of Ethics. *Australian Health Review, 45*(4), 398–406. doi: https://doi.org/10.1071/AH20215

National Aboriginal Community Controlled Health Organisation. (2022). *National Anti-Racism Framework: Submission to the Australian Human Rights Commission, February 2022.* https://www.naccho.org.au/app/uploads/2022/04/NACCHO-Submission-to-the-AHRC-Concept-Paper-for-a-National-Anti-Racism-Framework.pdf

Nursing and Midwifery Board of Australia. (2018). Cultural safety: Nurses and midwives leading the way for safer healthcare – Joint statement https://www.nursingmidwiferyboard.gov.au/codes-guidelines-statements/position-statements/leading-the-way.aspx

Rix, E., Doran, F., Wrigley, B. and Rotumah, D. (2024). Decolonisation for health: A life-long process of unlearning for Australian white nurse educators. *Nursing inquiry, 31*(2), p.e12616. doi: https://doi.org/10.1111/nin.12616

Sivertsen, N., Ryder, C. and Johnson, T. (2023). First Nations people often take on the 'cultural load' in their workplaces. Employers need to ease this burden. The Conversation. https://theconversation.com/first-nations-people-often-take-on-the-cultural-load-in-their-workplaces-employers-need-to-ease-this-burden-193858

Springall, T.L., Hall, K. and Carter, A.G. (2025). 'Mob aren't staying when there's no support': Enablers and barriers of recruitment and retention of First Nations midwifery students–A qualitative study. *Women and Birth, 38*(1), p. 101863. doi: https://doi.org/10.1016/j.wombi.2024.101863

Taylor, E.V., Lalovic, A. and Thompson, S.C. (2019). Beyond enrolments: a systematic review exploring the factors affecting the retention of Aboriginal and Torres Strait Islander health students in the tertiary education system. *International journal for equity in health, 18*(1), p. 136. doi: https://doi.org/10.1186/s12939-019-1038-7

Taylor, E.V., Lyford, M., Parsons, L., Mason, T., Sabesan, S. and Thompson, S.C. (2020). "We're very much part of the team here": A culture of respect for Indigenous health workforce transforms Indigenous health care. *PLoS One, 15*(9), p. e0239207. doi: https://doi.org/10.1371/journal.pone.0239207

Thackrah, R.D., Wood, J. and Thompson, S.C. (2021). Longitudinal follow up of early career midwives: insights related to racism show the need for increased commitment to cultural safety in Aboriginal maternity care. *International Journal of Environmental Research and Public Health, 18*(3), p. 1276. doi: https://doi.org/10.3390/ijerph18031276

Topp, S.M., Tully, J., Cummins, R., Graham, V., Yashadhana, A., Elliott, L. and Taylor, S. (2022). Rhetoric, reality and racism: the governance of Aboriginal and Torres Strait Islander health workers in a state government health service in Australia. *International journal of health policy and management, 11*(12), p. 2951. doi: https://doi.org/10.34172/ijhpm.2022.6750.

Uniting NSW.ACT (2025). First Nations People and Place Strategy Impact Report 2025.

West, R., Foster, K., Stewart, L. and Usher, K. (2016). Creating walking tracks to success: A narrative analysis of Australian Aboriginal and Torres Strait Islander nursing students' stories of success. *Collegian, 23*(4), pp. 349–354. doi: https://doi.org/10.1016/j.colegn.2016.08.001

10

EXPOSING COLONIALISM AND DEVELOPMENT OF ANTI-RACISM IN NURSING AND MIDWIFERY IN NIGERIA

Yetunde Akinnuoye

Introduction

This chapter investigates colonialism's historical and current effects on nursing and midwifery in Nigeria using comparative analysis from Ghana and Sierra Leone. It will examine how colonial influences shaped professional hierarchies, cultural factors in healthcare, and the ongoing fight for decolonising within the profession. This chapter will add to the conversation on how to develop a more equitable and culturally sensitive healthcare system in Africa by examining the enduring effects of colonialism and the current initiatives to combat racism and colonialism (Makhene, 2023). All national health systems depend on nursing and midwifery services. For generations, midwives and nurses have been delivering vital healthcare. In several nations across the world, they make up the bulk of the medical staff. The World Health Organization (WHO) has acknowledged its significance from its inception. Nigeria is situated in the tropical part of West Africa, comprises of different cultures with over 500 languages with multiple ethics groups.

The population of Nigeria is approximately 250 million. Nursing was recognised in 1949 in Nigeria. Thirty years later, by decree in 1979, midwifery was merged with the nursing council. A medical specialist that dates back to ancient times is midwifery. It may be considered to have evolved from the moment man got civilised enough to understand the delicate and complex nature of a woman's organs and reproductive process. Consequently, the custom of using a traditional birth attendant emerged at that time, although in its most basic shape and method. Anti-racism is the act of promoting equality and uprooting systemic racism within a group of people, culture, and society. Racism is the belief that one's own racialised group is inherently superior, often leading to prejudice, discrimination, or hostility toward others (Walker, 2022). Anti-colonialism is the concept of self-recognition

DOI: 10.4324/9781003565369-10

and belief, hence advocating for dismantling colonial powers and establishment. Colonialism: A system of control and exploitation where one nation dominates another, imposing its culture, language, and values (Watts, 1997).

Racism and coloniality are deeply rooted issues that affect many facets of Nigerian society, including the nursing and midwifery fields. These professions hold a unique position to influence both individual and community health outcomes, yet they are still caught up in systemic inequalities that have their roots in colonial history. Colonialism in Nigeria is a healthcare package that suits Western methods over local practices, leading to ongoing structural disparities. Moreover, systemic racism embedded in healthcare policies and institutions continues to disadvantage the less privileged groups of people, hindering the pursuit of fair healthcare access and delivery to Nigerians.

Colonialism's effects on nursing and midwifery go beyond historical accounts; they still have an impact on professional institutions, education, and legislation today, which sustain systemic and racial inequality (Zappas et al., 2021). The following paragraphs will purposely elaborate on anti-racism and anti-coloniality and their impacts within Nigeria's healthcare setting. By doing so, I will be able to analyse the historical contexts, assess current challenges, and suggest practical strategies that better suit our communities. Similarly, this book aims to uncover ways to benefit from anti-racism healthcare practices that tackle both cultural and systemic inequalities.

However, colonial legacies, which devalued and delegitimised Indigenous healthcare knowledge and cultural concerns while introducing Western medical methods as the right way, have had a profound impact on how these professions have developed in sub-Saharan Africa. Indigenous health systems in West Africa were reorganised by colonial governments, who ignored local knowledge and customs and imposed Eurocentric models that still have an impact on healthcare delivery, education, and professional hierarchies. In addition to upending the traditional roles of healers and birth attendants, the institutionalisation of Western medicine solidified gendered and racial inequalities that still exist today.

Nigeria's colonial government set up healthcare systems based on those of their European colonisers, especially Britain. Racialised hierarchies were established by the professionalisation of nursing and midwifery during colonial rule, frequently giving European-trained nurses positions of power over their African counterparts. Indigenous midwives and healers were marginalised by the institutionalisation of Western medical education and training, which resulted in the decline of culturally appropriate medical procedures that had supported African communities for many years (Zappas et al., 2021).

Different health leaders in Nigeria have questioned the dismantling of anti-racism and anti-coloniality. The initiatives aim to integrate Indigenous knowledge into healthcare education and practice, combat systemic injustice within the profession, and improve cultural humility. The chapter provides an opportunity to examine the extent to which anti-racist and anti-colonial frameworks are being utilised to improve nursing and midwifery education and practice. Therefore, to showcase this transparent case stories from within the sub-Saharan of Africa, the following countries—Nigeria, Ghana, and Sierra Leone are included in this review (Makhene, 2023).

How Nursing Profession Came to Be in Nigeria

Nursing has evolved, with its origins as a community service focused on maintaining health and providing support to the ill. Throughout history, nursing and medicine have been linked with the practice of nursing without medication during the Middle Ages. Nurses were viewed as inferior to religious authorities but later assisted doctors and priests in providing personal hygiene and custodial care. Christianity played a significant role in the growth of nursing practice, with the order of Deaconesses documenting its objectives. Women began entering nursing after Roman women's social standing improved by AD 300 (Arowolo, 2024). The number of women in nursing rose after the establishment of the Benedictine Order in the sixth century. The Crusades accelerated the growth of nursing and healthcare during the Middle Ages, establishing secular organisations like the Sisters of Charity in 1633.

Louise de Gras, a well-known widow, created the first educational initiative linked to a nursing order. This initiative covered both home visits and hospitalised patient care. Florence Nightingale, who enrolled with the Sisters of Charity in 1853, became the superintendent of the English General Hospitals in Turkey. She implemented significant changes to nursing practice, sanitation, and hygiene, helping the Barracks Hospital in Sentari, Turkey, lower its death rate from 42.7% to 2.2% in just six months (Arowolo, 2024).

Under Florence Nightingale's guidance, organised nursing began in the middle of the 1800s. Her nursing philosophy serves as the cornerstone of modern nursing practice. Her views on treating the ill were shaped by her nursing experience during the Crimean War and her religious values. She was educated at a higher socioeconomic level and had strong communication skills, as evidenced by her book "Notes on Nursing: What It Is and What It Is Not" and her numerous correspondences. She was able to handle politics and administration and travelled extensively.

Florence Nightingale has admirable traits—(see Chapter 1 of this book where this is also contested). She would be referred to as a statistician and epidemiologist in today's terms. She worked as a politician, a researcher, and a compassionate nurse to both the ill and the healthy. The evolving demands of society were mirrored in her nursing practice philosophy. Her understanding of how to prevent disease and how to recover from disease/ill health are explained in her notes on nursing from 1860 (Davies 2012, Turkowsi & Turkowski 2024) led her to believe that nursing should be have overall responsibility of a person's health. Florence may be considered an activist of some kind, given the position that women were supposed to play in her day. She saw the growth of nursing as a respectable earning career and constructive use of women's skills sets, and she was the one who strongly opposed the Victorian female role of indolence and marriage. She believed that in addition to compassion, activities should also be grounded on statistical data, observation and experience, dietary and sanitary expertise, and administrative abilities (Jones, 2000).

How Colonialism Embeds Racism in Nigeria Nursing Discipline

Nursing and midwifery were seen quite differently in the past than they are today. Even though nurses and the nursing profession are frequently discussed within their WHO publications from the 1940s and 1950s. Midwives are surprisingly under-represented as a separate group of health professionals in the 21st century. While the doctors are the first responder during emergency and nurses are qualified to give counsel to mothers about their pregnancy and birth outcomes. Consequently, in the 1960s, the WHO began to pay more attention to midwives and their abilities, significantly impacting mothers' and babies' health (Wolman et al., 1952). The findings from Wolman et al.'s (1952, p. 358) study say, "The fact that nursing job was perceived has a curative medicine, which are based on hospitalisation and have developed out of historical precedent in Western civilisations." Hence, this began the controversial discussion about the two disciplines.

The WHO established an Expert Committee on Nursing in 1950 and a Committee on Midwifery in 1954. Initially, nurses and midwives were seen as having different responsibilities, but their roles grew as the medical paradigm of care delivery was perceived as outdated. As the world's population expanded and people outlived their forebears, health services were needed to accommodate their evolving needs. The Expert Committee defined nursing service as providing care for illness prevention, health promotion, mental health and physical comfort, and care due to the patient's illness. However, the committee recognised the poor intake of both males and females in nursing. Nurses were considered more necessary than other health workers due to their direct, personal, and long-lasting patient interaction (WHO Expert Committee on Midwifery Training: first report, (Wolman et al., 1952).

The WHO Expert Committee on Midwifery Training's first meeting in The Hague in 1954 discussed the traditions, values, and customs of the people for whom midwifery services were to be provided in Nigeria. Education and awareness of women's cultural differences are key to their well-being, so the implementation was less successful. The meeting also recognised the need for those responsible for planning and overseeing maternity care services to have a comprehensive grasp of these aspects.

The three categories of midwifery staff covered to practice midwifery are the traditional birth attendant, the auxiliary midwife, and the fully trained midwife. Given that midwifery training was a nursing speciality in certain countries, midwifery training begins to grow in conjunction with the nursing curriculum.

The following definition of a midwife was accepted by the Expert Committee on Midwifery during its 1964 conference to address midwives in maternity care: "A midwife is a person who is qualified to practise midwifery." They are qualified to provide women with the care and guidance they require during their pregnancies, labours, and postpartum periods, to do regular births without supervision, and to attend to the needs of the newborn. They must always be able to spot the early warning symptoms of abnormal or possibly abnormal situations that call for a doctor's referral and be prepared to take immediate action without medical assistance. They could work in domiciliary services, hospitals, or health units. They have a significant role to play in community and family health education in each of these institutions. In some nations, their job also includes family planning, childcare, and gynaecology (Foucault, 1975).

As more individuals are attracted to the profession, the practitioners are becoming women's reproductive health experts in the safest possible clinical setting. Over time, it has become one of the most important professions in the wide range of healthcare delivery. The term "midwives" refers to both male and female midwifery practitioners. The word "midwife" comes from the words "mid" (with) and "wif" (woman). Midwives attend the baby's birth and provide prenatal care to expectant moms. They also offer the mother and the infant postpartum care (National Association of Nigeria nurses and midwives (NANNM), 2025).

The International Confederation of Midwives defines a midwife as an individual who has successfully finished the required course of study in midwifery and obtained the necessary credentials to be registered and/or legally licensed to practise midwifery. Often, they have been regularly admitted to a midwifery educational programme that is duly recognised in the nation in which they are situated. An apprenticeship is a conventional university programme, or a mix of the two might constitute an educational programme.

However, healthcare stakeholders, organisations, and specialists do not agree on this concept. For instance, although the WHO and the International Federation of Gynaecology and Obstetrics are credited with incorporating it into their policies and programmes, many medical professionals point out that it falls short in that it does not adequately address the traditional birth attendants who have been helping women give birth in most traditional settings worldwide, but particularly in developing nations, since ancient times. Aware of the delicate and vital nature of their work, midwives assist expectant mothers in getting the care, support, and guidance they need during pregnancy, delivery, and the postpartum phase. They perform deliveries and offer complete medical care for the newborn, including preventing neonatal complications, encouraging a healthy birth, identifying issues in both the mother and the child, obtaining medical or other necessary support, and performing emergency procedures (NANNM, 2025).

The following reasons impacted the evolution of nursing in Nigeria: world conflicts, religion, interprofessional communication, and British colonial administration. Historically, family members and women provided most of the care for the ill at home. The original communal structure did not include the idea of a nurse in the European sense. Families were seen to be responsible for caring for their members in good and bad health. However, midwife has always existed in all traditional communities. Traditional midwives who care for expectant mothers from conception until labour and delivery still exist in Nigeria. Both mother and newborn get postpartum care. The journey of nursing and midwifery dates back to 1933, with the Western curricula in place in Nigeria (Hargreaves, 1999).

Meanwhile, the colonial rules rejected the traditional cultures and classified their practices as non-scientifically correct. Thus, trained health professionals in Nigeria were employed in urban areas, leaving rural areas with healthcare staff deficits and struggling with health centres without equipment. Therefore, the people/communities resorted to Indigenous practices. The colonial impacts on Nigeria's healthcare systems are still visible in today's nursing and midwifery practices. Hence, in South Africa, the healthcare policies during apartheid entrenched racial inequalities, leaving a lasting mark on health outcomes. These challenges highlight the urgent need for anti-racism and anti-colonial initiatives within Nigeria's nursing and midwifery fields.

In the 19th century, missionaries from the United Kingdom came to Nigeria to evangelise, educate, and provide healthcare. As a result, the mission grounds house was the church, the school, and the clinic. Missionary nurses are graduates from Florence Nightingale School of Nursing or its curriculum. They mainly sought young men and women with just an elementary school education for on-the-job training in nursing procedures and abilities. Training in skills, from basic to advanced, was the primary focus (Brush, 1992).

The training was entirely task oriented. There was no central certification at first, as there were no structured courses. The missionary nursing sisters treated their disciples spiritually, psychologically, and physically, where the community's healthcare requirements were continuously evaluated, and suitable medical facilities were offered (Falola, 2025). The first group of nurses in the nation were those who received on-the-job training from missionary nursing sisters with training in the United Kingdom. These locally educated nursing staff members also embraced Christian principles and acted as evangelisation contacts in their communities. The two McCarter sisters facilitated mother and child health centres in Abeokuta and the surrounding areas.

While Mary Slessor was well-known in Calabar for her work with abandoned twins, Mary Slessor was a Scottish missionary who arrived in Nigeria in the late 19th century and became known for her humanitarian work, particularly in the Calabar region. Mary Slessor advocated for women's and children's rights and initiated the ending of the practice of killing twins in Nigeria. She worked extensively in healthcare and provided medical assistance to pregnant women during childbirth in rural areas. Though not a formally trained nurse or midwife, she was crucial in introducing Western medical interventions in maternal and infant care (Abdullahi, 2014).

Mary Slessor established the Western medicine curriculum in Nigeria and trained the local women in basic medical care and childbirth assistance. This is the genesis of midwifery practice, while postcolonial practice is the beginning of healthcare beyond traditional midwifery attendants. Her legacy contributed to the gradual recognition of women's roles in healthcare beyond traditional midwifery. However, her work also reflected the broader colonial influence that often-disregarded Indigenous medical knowledge in favour of Western practices. The legacy of Mary Slessor and other colonial healthcare interventions continues to shape contemporary nursing and midwifery in Nigeria. Some of the key impacts include the establishment of formal midwifery schools and standardised medical education, which initially marginalised traditional birth attendants but later sought to integrate community healthcare providers; the continued prioritisation of biomedical models over Indigenous health practices, leading to a lack of cultural responsiveness and humility in some aspects of maternal and child healthcare; the increasing role of women in nursing and midwifery leadership, reflecting the long-standing advocacy for women's rights and healthcare accessibility; Recent efforts to incorporate traditional and community-based healthcare approaches alongside formal nursing and midwifery education (Abdullahi, 2014).

Nigeria is characterised by remarkable linguistic and cultural diversity, with numerous languages and dialects spoken across its regions. This diversity posed significant challenges to early missionaries, particularly their limited understanding of local languages and their insufficient appreciation of the distinct cultural values, beliefs, and lifestyles of the people they sought to engage. Nevertheless, several pioneering efforts in linguistic development and literary production emerged through missionary work. For example, in Nigeria, one of the most enduring legacies of the Church Missionary Society (CMS) was the promotion of Yoruba literature. Bishop Samuel Ajayi Crowther, an indigenous scholar and missionary, produced the first translation of the Bible into Yoruba, a landmark achievement in African biblical scholarship. Furthermore, the publication of the first Yoruba newspaper, Iwe-Irohin, in 1859 marked a significant milestone in the development of African-language print culture. Comparable efforts were undertaken in other Nigerian languages, including Efik, Kanuri, and Igbo, thereby laying the foundation for indigenous literacy, literary traditions, and cultural preservation (Ezepue & Nwafor, 2023).

Missionaries demonstrated a strong commitment to learning local dialects, recognising that direct communication was more effective than reliance on interpreters for fostering genuine community understanding. In the context of Nigeria's multilingual landscape, this linguistic dedication extended beyond religious instruction to other aspects of social development, particularly healthcare. During the colonial era, missionaries played a pivotal role in shaping Nigeria's healthcare system. In order to effectively communicate medical procedures, hygienic practices, and preventive measures against diseases, they often relied on local intermediaries, including catechists and early Christian converts, who served as interpreters and translators. This strategy ensured that health-related knowledge was transmitted in culturally and linguistically accessible ways. Additionally, Pidgin English emerged as a practical lingua franca, enabling missionaries to reach diverse audiences across ethnic and linguistic boundaries.

Alongside hospitals and clinics, missionaries played a crucial role in developing the healthcare system in Nigeria. They set up schools and literacy initiatives to encourage literacy and increase access to medical knowledge. They translated medical brochures, hygiene manuals, and disease prevention materials into regional languages to raise public understanding of cleanliness and disease control. The training of native healthcare professionals was prioritised by missionaries, who set up official training programmes for regional medical assistants, nurses, and midwives. Another critical component of their approach to healthcare communication was cultural sensitivity. To reduce language barriers and customise healthcare services for particular populations, missionaries frequently founded regional missionary hospitals in linguistically homogenous areas. In addition to increasing access to healthcare, these initiatives established the groundwork for contemporary medical practice and education in Nigeria (Ezepue & Nwafor, 2023).

How Nigeria Nursing Has Started to Resist Colonialism in the Discipline

In Nigeria, the Royal Niger Company and the British colonial service initially provided medical care for their staff and families. Medical teams from the United Kingdom were deployed to oversee these services, and professional nurses trained in the United Kingdom formed an integral part of these teams. Two parallel healthcare systems subsequently emerged: one serving local Nigerians and the other serving colonial administrators.

During this period, hospitals were established across both Europe and Africa, where nursing sisters within the medical teams supervised and provided on-the-job training to local men and women. These trainees, who acquired practical skills but limited theoretical knowledge, became known as "probation nurses." Their training was based solely on the experiences of individual nursing sisters, as there was no standardised curriculum, regulatory oversight, or certification process (Ottuh, 2022).

Following the Second World War (ending in 1945), many Nigerian women with high school education travelled to the United Kingdom to pursue professional nursing training. Upon returning, most joined the Civil Service, though some struggled to apply their newly acquired skills in an often-unfriendly work environment. While some nurses left the profession, others remained and spearheaded reforms to elevate nursing education and practice in Nigeria. Among the pioneers were Adetoun Barley (later the first Nigerian Registrar of the Nursing Council), Francis Oguntolu (former Director of Nursing, Lagos University Teaching Hospital), Kofoworola Pratt (the first Nigerian Matron of University College Hospital, Ibadan), and Oluyinka Sofenwa (former Deputy Director of Nursing, University

College Hospital, Ibadan). Their collective efforts laid the foundation for professionalising nursing in the country (Ottuh, 2022).

The establishment of Nigeria's first Nursing Council and the appointment of an expatriate temporary Registrar in 1947 marked an important step in standard-setting. These reforms coincided with the political changes of the period, including constitutional reforms and negotiations for independence from Britain. Under the Richards Constitution, Nigeria was divided into three regions (East, West, and North) and the Federal Capital of Lagos. Alongside these political developments, schools of nursing were founded in Enugu, Ibadan, and Kaduna in 1949. These institutions were guided by structured curricula overseen by UK-trained nurses, though disparities persisted between state-led education and local communities (Arowolo, 2024).

The Health Policy of the time further mandated the sponsorship of high-achieving Nigerian boys and girls to study general nursing, midwifery, and specialised nursing in Great Britain. This represented a significant departure from earlier practices, where nursing trainees were often recruited after only six to eight years of elementary education. With this reform, students with solid secondary education backgrounds were encouraged to pursue nursing careers. By 1952, the policy had also established a school of nursing at the University College Hospital, Ibadan.

The Nightingale School of Nursing at St. Thomas' Hospital, London UK, provided the model for these developments, reinforcing the idea that nursing should attract well-educated candidates and be closely tied to professional and general education (Falola, 2025). These reforms reflected the government's determination to improve both the standards and public perception of nursing.

After the Nursing Council was formally established and empowered, it introduced minimum requirements for clinical teaching facilities, school curricula, and entry qualifications for student nurses. Nursing practice came under stronger regulation than midwifery, likely due to the more structured nature of nursing services compared with midwifery. A smaller proportion of highly trained professional nurses entered midwifery, and non-governmental organisations continued to exert considerable influence over midwifery practice (Zappas et al., 2021).

What More Needs to Be Done in Nigeria Nursing Profession and Education for Anti-Racism to Embed

According to Sheldon Watts, Western medicine not only failed to adequately treat the illnesses it helped create, but also became an instrument of imperialism (Kallaway, 2023). Sheryl Nestel expands on this perspective, arguing that "the motivations for colonial nurses were many, however, and all were deeply entangled in the politics of class, race, and gender" (Nestel, 1998). Anne McClintock further asserts that such narratives were used to justify "the imperialist violent enforcement of their [own] cultural and economic values," often by portraying Africa and Africans as "dirty," unclean, and lacking in well-ordered domesticity (McClintock and American Council of Learned Societies, 1995). The image of European nurses in immaculate uniforms, armed with carbolic bottles, was underpinned by the dismissal of African cleanliness and domestic practices.

These dynamics were not unique to Africa. Throughout the British Empire, nurses were deployed to evangelise the principles of "modern" nursing and sanitary reform (Sweet, 2004). Nestel (1998) describes the European nurse of the early 20th century as positioned at the intersection of race, class, and gender politics. She embodied middle-class hygienics against the "dirt" of Africa, modesty in contrast to constructed discourses of African female sexuality, and Christian medical science against what was framed as superstition.

The legacy of these historical injustices remains visible in Nigeria's present-day healthcare system. Poor infrastructure contributes significantly to the country's high maternal and fetal mortality rates. The African Population and Health Resource Center (APHRC) reports that Nigerian women face a one in 13 lifetime risk of dying in childbirth, with an estimated 40,000 maternal deaths annually, representing 14% of global maternal deaths (Nkomo, 2011). Disparities between urban and rural areas persist: while home births account for 35–37% of deliveries in urban settings, the figure rises to 75–90% in rural areas, often without the support of skilled attendants (Shilliam, 2010). Many rural women cite long distances and poor access to hospitals as barriers to care.

Colonial healthcare systems in Nigeria, Ghana, and Sierra Leone were largely modelled on British medical structures, often disregarding and displacing traditional African healing practices (Abdullahi, 2014). The institutionalisation of Western medical education marginalised indigenous healers and midwives, leading to the gradual erosion of culturally embedded practices that had sustained communities for generations. Traditional Birth Attendants (TBAs), who once played a vital role in maternal and neonatal care, were delegitimised by European-led medical organisations that positioned Western obstetrics and gynaecology as superior forms of knowledge and practice.

In light of this historical trajectory, there is a pressing need to reimagine healthcare education and delivery in ways that are anti-racist and anticolonial. This includes strengthening indigenous medical curricula, affirming the value of traditional knowledge systems, and fostering a more pluralistic approach to healthcare that respects and integrates local beliefs and practices alongside biomedical models.

Addressing health disparities requires an explicit recognition of racism and colonial legacies as critical social determinants of health. Nurses, in particular, hold both a moral and ethical responsibility to confront these inequities (Kimani, 2023). Combating racism in healthcare demands the implementation of anti-racist policies, the dismantling of discriminatory assumptions, e.g. the false narrative that Black women have a higher pain threshold (Hoffman et al. 2016), and the integration of historical, cultural, and political perspectives into nursing research and practice. Beyond documenting the harms caused by racism, scholars and practitioners must also interrogate how systemic oppression—including the enduring influence of colonialism—continues to shape health outcomes (Board on Health Sciences Policy, Institute of Medicine & Committee on Understanding and Eliminating Racial and Ethnic Disparities in Health Care 2002).

Western biomedical empiricism, which often privileges biological explanations while neglecting structural determinants of health, still dominates nursing education and practice. To redress this imbalance, international nursing education must expand discourses on diversity, equity, and inclusivity, while also acknowledging the power asymmetries embedded in global health partnerships and research. Strengthening collaborations with local researchers, practitioners, and communities is essential to ensuring that nursing scholarship is both contextually relevant and socially just (Kimani, 2023). As Zappas et al. (2021) remind us, although nursing is guided by the principle of non-maleficence ("do no harm"), systemic racism, unconscious bias, and social inequalities continue to perpetuate significant harm across patient populations, families, and communities. Thus, nursing as a profession bears a responsibility—rooted in ethics and social justice—to actively work toward dismantling racism and advancing health equity.

In the Nigerian context, nurses and midwives face acute challenges, including workforce depletion, inadequate training opportunities, and limited institutional support. Many healthcare professionals emigrate in search of better working conditions, a phenomenon exacerbated by the government's persistent neglect of both healthcare training and practice. Consequently, political leaders and elites often seek medical treatment abroad, particularly in Western countries such as the United Kingdom and the United States, reflecting a lack of sustained investment in domestic health systems. To reverse this trend, Nigerian leadership must prioritise healthcare as a national imperative, making it central to policy agendas and urgently enacting reforms to strengthen local capacity, retain skilled professionals, and ensure equitable access to quality healthcare.

Decolonising the nursing curriculum is an essential step toward achieving equity. Since Florence Nightingale's Victorian-era influence, the nursing curriculum has remained largely Western-centric, often sidelining African epistemologies. Anti-racism requires embedding African scholars' contributions and lived experiences into the curriculum, rather than relegating them to elective or peripheral modules. Ezepue and Nwafor (2023) argue that second-generation colonialism functioned by controlling knowledge systems—through science, law, economics, and health—while first-generation colonialism targeted geographical and physical domination (Makhene, 2023). Neo-colonialism, therefore, reflects a state in which political independence coexists with continued intellectual and economic subordination. Anti-racism, in its simplest form, is the undoing of this process (Makhene, 2023).

The Covid-19 pandemic highlighted the fragility of resource-dependent systems and reinforced the urgency of curriculum reform in the 21st century and the Fourth Industrial Revolution. An anti-racism nursing curriculum must challenge colonial epistemologies, integrate local and indigenous knowledge, and prepare nurses to address structural determinants of health. It needs to be policy-driven to start the change, so we need nurse and midwifery activist lobbying government and regulatory bodies. Only through such transformation can nursing education in Africa advance towards equity, inclusivity, justness, and global relevance.

The sustainability of the profession in Nigeria, however, remains under serious threat. Many nurses and midwives have emigrated due to poor remuneration and limited opportunities. On average, a nurse or midwife in Nigeria earns less than £100 per month, while facing overwhelming caseloads, with ratios as stark as one nurse per 100,000 patients and one midwife per 364 women. These alarming figures underscore the urgency of the United Nations' 2015 call for healthcare to become a government priority in Nigeria.

Currently, Nigeria has approximately 3,605 hospitals (both public and private) to serve a population of over 250 million people. This gross imbalance between healthcare infrastructure and population demand contributes significantly to the nation's high mortality rate and low life expectancy, currently at 53 years. Moving forward, Nigeria must invest in establishing more healthcare facilities, improving healthcare delivery systems, and ensuring fair and competitive salaries for nurses and midwives. Strengthening the nursing and midwifery workforce is not only a matter of professional sustainability but also a critical determinant of the nation's overall health outcomes (Williams et al. 2014).

Conclusion

Nursing education in Nigeria has been significantly influenced by advancements in the United Kingdom and the United States. Florence Nightingale's universal definition of nursing, which emphasises the application of natural laws to promote health and facilitate recovery from illness, remains a foundational concept in nursing practice. Today, nurses and midwives worldwide utilise various communication channels, including printed resources, electronic materials, and online platforms, to address pressing global health issues. Organisations such as the International Council of Nurses (ICN) and the West African College of Nursing (WACN) exemplify efforts to promote globalisation and collaboration within the nursing and midwifery professions.

A historical review highlights the importance of anti-colonialist and anti-racist movements in Nigeria and across Africa. The legacy of colonialism and the experiences of racism, particularly among healthcare professionals in the diaspora, have deeply influenced the structure of nursing education and the ways in which nurses apply their training in patient care. The Global Strategy on Human Resources for Health: Workforce 2030 recognises the critical role of nursing and midwifery in meeting population health needs. Achieving this vision requires efficient utilisation of scarce resources, implementation of evidence-based workforce policies, and enforcement of robust regulatory frameworks. Furthermore, fostering a diverse skill mix, ensuring safe and supportive working conditions, promoting continuous professional development, and establishing clear career pathways are essential for advancing the profession.

The future prosperity of nursing and midwifery in Nigeria is closely tied to socioeconomic empowerment. Real progress demands stronger political will from health planners and policymakers to design and implement initiatives that cultivate anti-racism leadership within the profession. Nurses and midwives must increasingly be included in policy formulation and decision-making processes, ensuring that their expertise shapes healthcare strategies at both national and international levels. Policy advocacy efforts must be reinforced through both new and existing initiatives that prioritise anti-racism leadership development in nursing and midwifery.

Reflective Activity

Having read the chapter, we invite you to reflect on your key learning and its implications for your professional practice as a nurse or midwife using Bain et al.'s (2002) 5R framework (pp. 13–15):

- Reporting—what is it in your situation you want to transform after reading this chapter?
- Responding—what are your personal observations regarding your own situation/context in relation to what is raised in this chapter?
- Relating—what is/are the theoretical/research/data/legislative, etc. understandings relationship to under consideration in this chapter that you could apply to your situation/context?
- Reasoning—Identify how the chapter findings matter to your situation/context and how will you interrogate your situation/context and what will help you from this chapter.
- Reconstructing—Identify your action plans to reframe and rebuild a transformative way forward to change from the situation in your context.

References

Abdullahi, A.A. (2014). Trends and challenges of traditional medicine in Africa. *African journal of traditional, complementary, and alternative medicines*, *8*(5 Suppl), 115–123. DOI: 10.4314/ajtcam.v8i5S.5.

Arowolo, D.E. (2024). Dancing on a knife-edge: European colonisation of Africa and Nigeria's cultural crisis. *African identities*, *22*(2), 430–446. DOI: 10.1080/14725843.2022.2040422.

Bain, J.D., Ballantyne, R., Mills, C. and Lester, N.C. (2002). *Reflecting on practice: Students teachers' perspectives*. Post Pressed.

Board on Health Sciences Policy, Institute of Medicine & Committee on Understanding and Eliminating Racial and Ethnic Disparities in Health Care. (2002). *Unequal treatment: Confronting racial and ethnic disparities in health care*. National Academies Press.

Brush, L.D. (1992). Endless crusade: Women social scientists and progressive reform. Ellen Fitzpatrick Lady Bountiful revisited: Women, philanthropy, and power. Kathleen D.

Muncy, R. (1991; online edn, Oxford Academic, 31 Oct. 2023). Creating a female dominion in American Reform 1890–1935. *Signs: Journal of women in culture and society, 17*(4), 829–834. DOI: 10.1093/oso/9780195057027.001.0001.
Davies R. (2012). 'Notes on nursing: what it is and what it is not'. (1860): by Florence Nightingale. *Nurse education today, 32*(6), 624–626. https://doi.org/10.1016/j.nedt.2012.04.025
Ezepue, E.M. and Nwafor, C.G. (2023). October 1: Metaphorizing Nigeria's collective trauma of colonization. *SAGE open, 13*(3). DOI: 10.1177/21582440231197271.
Falola, T. (2025). *Understanding colonial Nigeria: British rule and its impact.* Cambridge University Press.
Foucault, M. (1975). The birth of the clinic. An archaeology of medical perception. *Medical history, 19*(4), 405–406. DOI: 10.1017/S0025727300020585 (translated from the French by A. M. Sheridan Smith).
Hargreaves, J.D. (1999). [Chapter review] Raymond F. Betts, "Decolonization". *Journal of African history, 40*(3), 518. https://go.exlibris.link/bbNSs4pp
Hoffman, K.M., Trawalter, S., Axt, J.R. and Oliver, M.N. (2016). Racial bias in pain assessment and treatment recommendations, and false beliefs about biological differences between blacks and whites. *Proceedings of the national academy of sciences - PNAS, 113*(16), 4296–4301. DOI: 10.1073/pnas.1516047113.
Jones, C. (2000). Levels of racism: A theoretic framework and a gardener's tale. *American journal of public health (1971), 90*(8), 1212–1215. DOI: 10.2105/AJPH.90.8.1212.
Kallaway, P. (2023). The changing face of colonial education in Africa: Education, science and development. *African studies review, 66*(1), 237–239. https://go.exlibris.link/JqCXsSWh
Kimani, R.W. (2023). Racism, colonialism and the implications for nursing scholarship: A discussion paper. *Journal of advanced nursing, 79*(5), 1745–1753. DOI: 10.1111/jan.15634.
MacLean, L.M. (2017). Neoliberal democratisation, colonial legacies and the rise of the non-state provision of social welfare in West Africa. *Review of African political economy, 44*(153), 358–380. DOI: 10.1080/03056244.2017.1319806.
Makhene, A. (2023). Decolonisation of the nursing education curriculum in Gauteng province, South Africa: A concept analysis. *Health SA = SA* Gesondheid, *28*(1), 2449–2449. DOI: 10.4102/hsag.v28i0.2449.
McClintock, A. and American Council of Learned Societies. (1995). *Imperial leather: Race, gender, and sexuality in the colonial contest*, 1st edn., Routledge.
National association of Nigeria nurses and midwives (NANNM). (2025). *Midwifery & Midwives*. https://nannm.com.ng/
Nestel, S. (1998). (Ad)ministering angels: Colonial nursing and the extension of empire in Africa. *The Journal of medical humanities, 19*(4), 257–277. DOI: 10.1023/A:1024908110021.
Nkomo, S.M. (2011). A postcolonial and anti-colonial reading of 'African' leadership and management in organization studies: Tensions, contradictions and possibilities. *Organization (London, England), 18*(3), 365–386. DOI: 10.1177/1350508411398731.
Ottuh, J.A. (2022). The 3Cs of Colonisation and their impacts on African Slavery: The Nigeria's experience. *Black theology an international journal, 20*(1), 41–65. DOI: 10.1080/14769948.2022.2038909.
Shilliam, R. (2010). *International relations and non-Western thought: Imperialism, colonialism and investigations of global modernity.* Routledge.
Sweet, H. (2004). 'Wanted: 16 nurses of the better educated type': provision of nurses to South Africa in the late nineteenth and early twentieth centuries. *Nursing inquiry, 11*(3), 176–184. DOI: 10.1111/j.1440-1800.2004.00228.x.
Turkowski, Y. and Turkowski, V. (2024). Florence Nightingale (1820–1910): The founder of modern nursing. *Curēus (Palo Alto, CA), 16*(8), e66192. DOI: 10.7759/cureus.66192.

Walker, B.B. (2022). The colonial foundations of global health: Britain, Gold Coast, and Ghana, 1919–61. In *Religion in Global Health and Development: The case of twentieth century Ghana*. McGill-Queen's University Press (pp. 29–75).

Watts, S.J. (1997). *Epidemics and history: Disease, power, and imperialism*. Yale University Press.

Williams, S.D., Hansen, K., Smithey, M., Burnley, J., Koplitz, M., Koyama, K., Young, J. and Bakos, A. (2014). Using social determinants of health to link health, workforce diversity, care quality and access, and health disparities to achieve health equity in nursing. *Public health reports (1974)*, *129*(1_suppl2), 32–36. DOI: 10.1177/00333549141291S207.

Wolman, A., Waksman, S.A., Workman, W.G., Steele, J.H., Petry, L., Eddy, N.B., Stowman, K., Coatney, G.R., Dunn, H.L., Eastman, N.J., Miller, L.C., Menninger, W.C., Mahoney, J.F., Hundley, J.M., Nyswander, D.B., Dunham, E.C., Hiscock, I.V. and Hilleboe, H.E. (1952). The work of the World Health Organization expert committees. *Public Health Reports (1896)*, *67*(4), 358–369. DOI: 10.2307/4588080.

Zappas, M., Walton-Moss, B., Sanchez, C., Hildebrand, J.A. and Kirkland, T. (2021). The decolonization of nursing education. *Journal for nurse practitioners*, *17*(2), 225–229. DOI: 10.1016/j.nurpra.2020.11.006.

11

THE INVISIBLE RACISM; RACISM AGAINST GYPSY, ROMA, TRAVELLERS AND STRATEGIES FOR IMPROVED NURSING AND MIDWIFERY PROVISION

Vanessa Heaslip and Hal King

Introduction

The purpose of this chapter is to introduce readers to the hidden racism experienced by Gypsy, Roma, Travellers (GRT). It commences by providing a clear definition of who GRT are and their numbers within the United Kingdom (UK). It continues by discussing how racism against members of these communities is linked to anti-Gypsyism[1] movement which has been prevalent since the 14th and 15th centuries which has continued. Furthermore, contemporary racism experienced by GRT is explored by examining their invisibilisation in data collection at national and international levels, their experiences of discrimination and hate crime internationally, before examining health inequities fuelled by anti-Gypsyism in the UK and across Europe. The chapter concludes by exploring healthcare experiences of GRT and the roles of nurses and midwives in promoting culturally safe care and inviting readers to reflect upon their personal values and professional practice when working with GRT.

Background and Historical Context

GRT[2] is an umbrella term used to denote different GRT minoritised ethnic communities including Romany Gypsies, Irish Travellers, Welsh Gypsies, Eastern and European Roma (Heaslip et al., 2016). Whilst Roma is an umbrella term which includes Sinti, Kale, Manus, Kalderas, Lovari and Romanichals (James, 2021). Whilst in this chapter we use the umbrella term GRT, it is important to note that each minoritised ethnic group is separate and has distinct cultural values.

Romany Gypsies and European Roma share a common ancestry, dating back approximately 1,500 years to Northern India, evidenced by both genetic and

DOI: 10.4324/9781003565369-11

philological records (Friends, Families and Travellers (FFT), n.d.; 2). Irish Travellers are a distinctive indigenous minoritised ethnic group native to Ireland (Irish Traveller Movement, 2019) but share a rich cultural history of nomadism. Some GRT remain nomadic, moving from place to place, however, legislative changes (Section 60C of the Criminal Justice and Public Order Act, 1994 (Legislation.Gov.UK, 2026)) make trespassing with an intent to reside in a vehicle a criminal offence (FFT, 2024a), which have impacted upon this free movement. As a result, GRT live in a range of accommodation including houses, local authority Gypsy, Traveller sites, privately owned sites, chalets on private land and very few remain mobile, living on transit sites or the side of the road. The most recent government caravan count in England estimates 27,273 Gypsy, Traveller caravans (Gov.UK, 2025). Despite this increasingly settled status, James (2021; 149) argues there remains a cultural nomadism in their predisposition to think and act in a boundless fashion, linked to notions of freedom and autonomy, living in close groups with strong bonds of familiar attachment and strict moral codes.

The history of racialised oppression against GRT is contingent on the respective minoritised ethnic group. However, discrimination is rooted in an 'anti-Gypsyism' sentiment stemming from the Middle Ages. Romani people began travelling through Europe during the 14th and 15th centuries, arriving in England in the 16th century, where they were identified by a 'misnomer', when mistaken as Egyptians, they were labelled 'Gypsies' (Sierra, 2024; 13). This term was not intended originally as a pejorative term but later became so across Europe and Ireland. Whilst some GRT find the term offensive, others, particularly Romany Gypsies in England, have reclaimed the term. It is important to note that many Irish Travellers find the term Gypsy to be highly offensive, preferring that the term Traveller is used.

The animosity and prejudice towards GRT and nomadism broadly speaking can be seen mutilating throughout history, reaching the height of its depravity in the 20th century with the Holocaust and Romani genocide, referred to as 'Porajmos', a Roma word for 'devouring' (FFT, 2024a; 3). Sierra (2024) argues the nature of events such as the Romani Holocaust can only be made sense of 'if set into the historic background of anti-Gypsyism, a complex bias as long-running as the very history of the Roma people in the Western world' (Sierra, 2024; 13). It is estimated that 500,000 Roma and Sinti were killed during the Holocaust, something that is sadly little invoked or indeed known by the general public. This ignorance is attested by YouGov research in 2019, which revealed that '55% of British adults surveyed' were unaware of the Roma and Sinti Holocaust (FFT, 2024a; 1).

Anti-Gypsyism remains today despite some GRT communities (Romany, Scottish Gypsies/Travellers and Irish Travellers) protection as a racialised group in the 2010 Equality Act (Legislation.gov.uk, n.d.). This Act prohibits discrimination, harassment and victimisation of a variety of protected characteristic groups, of which one, is race. The chapter will now explore the variety of different ways in which GRTs' experience racism as well as suggest ways forward to ameliorate this.

Invisibilisation of Gypsy, Roma, Travellers

It is difficult to estimate the true numbers of GRT globally as many countries do not collate data on these minoritised ethnic communities. The most recent estimate across Europe is 10–12 million (European Commission, 2020), however, this figure is based upon estimates from 2012, some 13 years ago. Indeed, in the UK it was only in the 2011 census that Gypsy or Irish Traveller was first introduced, and not until the 2021 census Roma was added as a minoritised ethnic category. According to the most recent census in the UK undertaken in 2021/2022 (UK Parliament, 2024) there were 77,340 people identifying with Gypsy and Traveller ethnic groups and 107,800 identifying as Roma (see Table 11.1). Whilst minoritised ethnic identity is important to GRT sense of self (Borkowska et al., 2023), many charities argue that due to the huge void of trust between the state, public services and people from these communities (Traveller Movement, 2022) very few GRT identify themselves in state and public records. As such, they argue that these numbers are likely to be a small fraction of the actual numbers (Kirkby et al., 2023; Traveller Movement, 2022). Furthermore, research by Brown et al. (2013) estimated that the population of GRT in the UK in 2012 was more likely to be between 400,000–500,000 and we argue with migration and population changes, that it is likely to be considerably higher in 2025.

This invisibilisation of GRT within official statistics we assert is a form of institutional racism which seeks to 'hide' the existence of GRT. Invisibilisation, a process of oppression, refers to the way language and imagery promote individuals and groups in strong positions whilst rendering others 'invisible' (Thompson, 2011). Ryden (2013) developed this notion further to also include actions, beliefs and discourses. The fact that despite the hundreds of centuries that GRT have been in existence that their inclusion in official statistics is only recent or completely missing highlights their invisibilisation. McDonald and Wingfield (2008) explored this notion of invisibility within institutional racism highlighting the 'organisational habitus' that occurs due to the norms, practices and culture of historically predominantly white institutions that reinforce racial and ethnic inequity. The paradox here is that GRT fall within white ethnicity, however categorising 'white' ethnicity fails to capture the different experiences of a variety of different minoritised

TABLE 11.1 Numbers of Gypsy, Roma, Travellers in the UK (UK Parliament, 2024)

County	*Numbers*
England and Wales	• 71,440 (0.12% of the population) identified as a Gypsy or Irish Traveller • 103,100 (0.2% of the population) identified as Roma
Northern Ireland	• 2,600 (0.1% of the population) identified as Irish Traveller • 1,500 (0.1% of the population) identified as Roma
Scotland	• 3,300 (0.1% of the population) identified as a Gypsy or Traveller • 3,200 (0.1% of the population) identified as Roma

ethnic groups such as, but not exclusively, Gypsy Roma, Travellers. This invisibilisation then fails to capture the frequent deleterious consequences faced by these racialised and minoritised ethnic groups (McDonald and Wingfield, 2008; 29) as well as rendering them 'the other'. This othering of GRT (more on this later) perpetuates the feeling of difference and distrust in the state and official organisations by members of these communities who in turn feel they have little choice but to hide their ethnicity for safety and self-preservation, further promoting their invisibilisation in official statistics.

Racism towards Gypsy, Roma, Travellers

The Eurobarometer on discrimination in the European Union (EU) noted that 65% of EU citizens recognise that discrimination against Roma is widespread (EU, 2023), a rise from 61% in 2019 (EU, 2019). In the UK, research by the Traveller Movement (2017) with 214 GRT identified that 91% of respondents experienced discrimination because of their ethnicity, and a further 77% experienced hate speech or a hate crime. Furthermore, research by the Equality and Human Rights Commission (2018) noted that across the different protected characteristic groups, GRT were the only group for which the most frequent response was a negative perception (44%), and this was followed by immigrants (27%), Muslims (22%) and Black people (5%). This research highlights the stark contrast and the apparent 'acceptability' of racism towards GRT that we wish to explore in more detail.

Tremlett (2023) argues there is a normalisation of racism of GRT and this can be seen in research conducted by Thompson and Woodger (2020) on hate crime. Their research examined 115 cases reported to the Report Racism GRT website which included online hate (67% of cases) including social media abuse, intimidation, harassment and violence. Online comments on Facebook included responses such as 'Go and commit suicide' and 'Go hang yourself' (Thompson and Woodger, 2020; 52) but these responses were seen somehow as acceptable by fellow users. Interestingly only 20% of these cases were reported to police, and of these only 18% was reported from the communities themselves and the most common reason for lack of reporting was a lack of confidence the police would act (Thompson and Woodger, 2020). This fear of being treated unfairly by the police was also reported in wider research undertaken by the Office for National Statistics (ONS) (2022a). Within GRT communities there is an acknowledgement that there appears to be different rules regarding racism for them as GRT and for other minoritised ethnic groups (Heaslip, 2015; 134)

> *I mean, if it was a Black man, they couldn't say 'No Blacks', could they? ...they wouldn't be able to say to them what they say to us and get away with it, or any other ethnic minority. They just wouldn't get away with it. They'd get locked up. But it's alright for them to do it to us*
>
> *—Johnny (Romany Gypsy)*

Garner (2017) argues, and we concur, that in understandings of racism there is blind spot in relation to GRT and a perception that the negative attitudes towards GRT cannot be racism if it is perpetuated 'white upon white'. Yet he highlights that race is both a political and social construct that includes bodies and culture within a hierarchical and analytical frame to generate and reflect power relationships (Garner, 2017). In this way, racism can be argued to be beyond just skin colour. Bhopal and Myers (2008) develop this notion further and refer to the 'outsiders to established whiteness' where they feel GRT locate.[3] In this they note whiteness to be beyond simple skin colour to include background and ethnicity (thereby culture), in which GRT fall within the category of a 'white outsider'. In which they are somehow an undesirable white community, leading to their othering and exclusion. This can be understood further using Hutchison et al. (2018) adaptation of Intergroup Threats (ITT) developed by Stephan et al. (2009). The framework notes both realistic and symbolic threats perceived by one group (ingroup) to another (outgroup), see Figure 11.1.

Hutchison et al. (2018) used this framework to explore public attitudes (n=180) towards Gypsies and Travellers in the UK, which identified an overall negative attitude towards Gypsies and Travellers. Figure 11.1 identifies how perceptions of GRT, as criminal, deviant, dishonest people (realistic threat) who had different beliefs, morals and norms (symbolic threat) pose a threat to wider society. This research highlighted a correlation between perceived realistic and symbolic threats

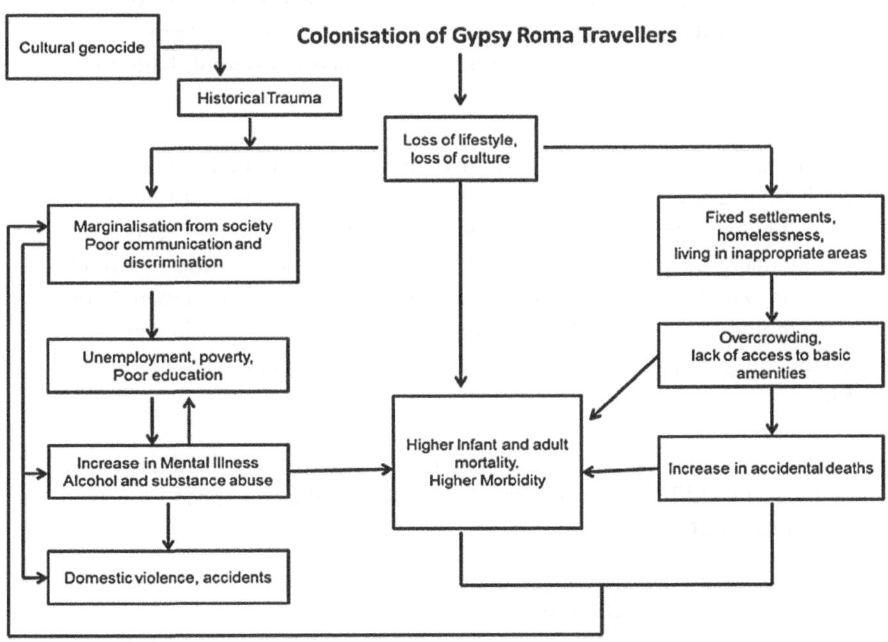

FIGURE 11.1 Intergroup Threats and Gypsies and Travellers

Sources: Adapted from Hutchison et al., 2018.

and negative attitudes towards Gypsies and Travellers (Hutchison et al., 2018). It is this anti-Gypsyism that is the root cause of GRT exclusion manifested through racism, discrimination, prejudice, stereotypes, stigmatisation, hate speech and hate crime (European Union, 2024).

The result of anti-Gypsyism is 'othering' of the community. Othering is essentially a process whereby there becomes a distinction between the majority group and those who are minoritised, who are designated as unwelcome outsiders. Ahmed (2006) identified that racialisation encompasses a sense of belonging, a feeling of being at home within a geographical space, therefore any consideration of racism must also consider the degree to which individuals are made (or not) to feel welcome. Schwalbe et al. (2000) identified different types of othering including oppressive othering, where one group seeks advantage by defining the other group as morally and/or intellectually inferior, and implicit othering by creation of powerful selves where the majority group see themselves as powerful and worthy, therefore anyone not like them must be unpowerful or unworthy. Heaslip (2015; 144) doctoral research thesis highlighted the impact of this othering of GRT on their vulnerability, highlighting this othering denoted them an almost 'unhuman state' (see below) where they were not afforded the same rights as their fellow human beings.

> I am located in the world, but I do not feel part of it. Instead, I sit on the periphery both physically, socially and psychologically, hidden from view. People do not want to see me, nor do they accept who I am. Instead, they want me to be different… but in being different, I am not me.
>
> I feel trapped, I cannot live the life I wish to live, a life thousands before me have lived, yet I am told that this way of life is wrong, but I have no voice to challenge because no one wants to listen, and no one hears.
> I am vulnerable because I cannot be me, I cannot live my life as I would wish, instead I am dictated to by others, others who do not know me nor wish to understand me. I feel as though I have to beg to be allowed to do the things that are important to me, why should that be, I am human too.
>
> I am dying, in the future there will be none of me, yet my death is slow and painful and I weep and grieve for the loss of the life I have known, that others will never see.

Health, Healthcare and Racism

Having articulated the experiences, discrimination and racism faced by GRT in the UK and Europe, it is therefore unsurprising that this has implications on their health and well-being. Life expectancy for Roma across Europe is less than the general population; for Roma women it is 11 years less and for Roma men 9.1 years less (European Union Agency for Fundamental Human Rights, 2021). In the UK, there is also a reduction in life expectancy for GRT, including a 7.1 reduction in life expectancy for women and a 10.3-year reduction for men (European Union Agency for Fundamental Human Rights, 2020). Factors affecting this reduced life expectancy are multifactorial and Heaslip et al. (2019a) argue that much of this is linked to colonisation and their marginalised status (see Figure 11.2).

Starting with accommodation (Figure 11.2) many GRT live in substandard accommodation. Research by the European Union Agency for Fundamental Human Rights (2020) noted that 20% of Roma and Traveller households are affected by environmental problems (pollution, grime, smoke, dust, unpleasant smells or polluted water). This rises to 25% for those living on official GRT sites and 26% for those living in caravans (European Union Agency for Fundamental Human Rights, 2020). This occurs largely due to anti-Gypsyism, reflected in the multiple protests on the development of GRT sites within local communities resulting them being located inhospitable areas such as near main roads, quarries, etc. This, Bloch and Quarmby (2024) argue, is a form of environment racism as it exposes minoritised communities (in this case GRT) to disproportionate levels of environment harm. This results in an increase in respiratory illness (Anastasaki et al., 2022) and

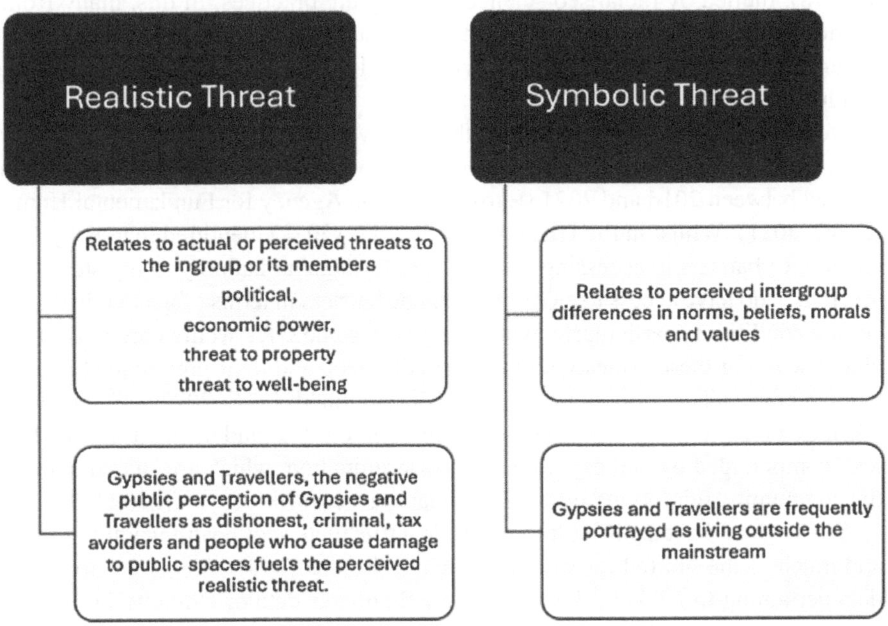

FIGURE 11.2 Colonisation of Gypsy, Roma, Travellers (Cunningham and Stanley, 2003)

Sources: Adapted by Heaslip et al. (2019a).

accidental deaths (Abdalla et al., 2013). This coupled with issues related to the extreme marginalisation and discrimination that GRT face (Figure 11.2) impacting upon their wider social determinants of health including poorer educational attainment and difficulty securing employment (ONS, 2022b). Furthermore, research by Greenfields and Rogers (2020; 14) on the psychological effects of hate crime of GRT communities identified the '*persistent and demoralising effect of the hate speech and discrimination*'. In addition, colonisation experienced by GRT in that they are expected to confirm to the majority culture, results in poor mental health and increased suicidality (Dagli and Webb, 2025). These negative spirals culminate in higher mortality and morbidity experienced by GRT.

It is also important to recognise the impact of intersectionality within GRT communities. Corradi (2021) argues that GRT women across Europe experience multiple discriminations linked to patriarchy, anti-Gypsism and extreme poverty, which perpetuates health inequity. In terms of maternal health, there is further evidence of inequity, racism and discrimination. O'Brien et al. (2024) systematic review on pregnancy outcomes in GRT communities identified increased risk of congenital abnormalities, growth restriction, premature birth, perinatal and early childhood mortality (O'Brien et al., 2024). Furthermore, a review of enforced sterilisations across Europe by Rowlands et al. (2024) identified widespread sterilisation campaigns on GRT as late as in the early 1990s (with the last alleged case occurring in 2018), fuelled by racialised science and eugenic practices. In this, many Roma women were sterilised without their informed consent or coerced into sterilisation under threat of loss of employment, withdrawal of welfare or removal of existing children (Rowlands et al., 2024).

Despite the well-known global health inequity experienced by GRT, the numbers of Roma experiencing discrimination in accessing healthcare across Europe has increased between 2016 and 2021 (European Union Agency for Fundamental Human Rights, 2021). Whilst in the UK, research by FFT (2022) identified that many GRT experience barriers in accessing primary care through an inability to register with a GP. If they do have access to a GP, there can be barriers in terms of gender, in that for certain conditions (particularly gynaecological), some GRT women are uncomfortable discussing these issues with male practitioners, and their preference to have a women practitioner is often not respected or facilitated (ONS, 2022c). Work undertaken by FFT (2023) on maternal health highlighted 'fear and mistrust of state bodies', compounded by bad experiences of discrimination, which are shared amongst the community, reinforcing evasion of engaging with services (FFT, 2023; 36).

Within the UK, it is difficult to ascertain a true picture of health inequity of GRT and much of the limited research is quite old (before 2010). This is due to limited data pertaining to GRT. In the UK, the NHS collates data of ethnicity in the NHS Data Dictionary (NHS England, 2022), recognising the importance of collating ethnicity data to understand the inequalities faced by different ethnic groups. Despite this recognition, there remains an invisibility of data pertaining to GRT health experiences as the NHS Data Dictionary ethnicity criteria does not include GRT as a distinct minoritised ethnic category (Table 11.2), despite calls from charities to

TABLE 11.2 NHS Data Dictionary (NHS England, 2022)

National Code	*National Code Definition*
A	White – British
B	White – Irish
C	White – Any other White background
D	Mixed – White and Black Caribbean
E	Mixed – White and Black African
F	Mixed – White and Asian
G	Mixed – Any other mixed background
H	Asian or Asian British – Indian
J	Asian or Asian British – Pakistani
K	Asian or Asian British – Bangladeshi
L	Asian or Asian British – Any other Asian background
M	Black or Black British – Caribbean
N	Black or Black British – African
P	Black or Black British – Any other Black background
R	Other Ethnic Groups – Chinese
S	Other Ethnic Groups – Any other ethnic group
Z	Not stated
99	Not known

address this. This invisibilisation as discussed earlier is a form of institutional racism, as GRT are subsumed into the White category, despite other minoritised ethnic groups being sub-categorised.

Nurses and midwives are the largest healthcare professional group, responsible for 90% of care delivered (World Health Organization, 2021), and as such could do much to address health inequity and the poor experiences of healthcare experienced by GRT. Indeed, both the International Council of Nurses (2021) and the Nursing and Midwifery Council (NMC) (2018) codes of ethics highlight the importance of nurses upholding individual human rights and practising in ways which promotes diversity, although the NMC is not as explicit regarding the promotion of cultural safety. Despite this, research by Heaslip et al. (2019b) with n=23 student nurses from four European countries (UK, Spain, Belgium, Turkey) identified that despite limited formal contact with GRT communities most students had negative perceptions of working with them due to perceptions related to aggression, violence and criminal activities. In terms of midwifery, O'Brien et al. (2024) systematic review on pregnancy outcomes in GRT communities identified racism was a barrier to care. Again, there is a perception within the communities that racism by healthcare practitioners is somehow not perceived as racism, nor would these practitioners treat other minoritised ethnic groups the same way

> *...like, a Muslim family come in, and they pretty much lived in the hospital, and they didn't get talked about as much as...because of their fear of racism and stuff. But they didn't get talked as much as Travellers do. Funny old world*
>
> *—Layla (Irish Traveller). (Heaslip, 2015; 134)*

> *When I had my first miscarriage, I was living roadside with very little understanding of what was happening to me. I couldn't get a midwife to come to the site and had no access to toilets or shower…*
>
> *(FFT, 2023; 48)*

Anecdotal experiences of talking to nurses and midwives have highlighted that when treating GRT they will often go in pairs to provide care (even though this is not routine practice) due to fear of working with the community because of perceptions of aggression and violence. These perceptions (or worldviews) are developed from childhood experiences, societal norms and wider media representations. Worldviews are defined by Wilson et al. (2018; 3812) as

> *…ways of experiencing and thinking about the world we live in, evident in commonly agreed beliefs and practices held by people belonging to particular groups*

It is important to recognise that nurses and midwives have their own worldviews (personal and professional), which will influence the way they engage with patients, their families, communities and other health and social care practitioners. It is also important to recognise that patients/service users will also have their own worldviews, and these may not be the same as the nurses and midwives looking after them. An example of contrasting worldviews in the care of GRT is evident in end-of-life care. GRT have a very strong family culture, often living alongside extended families, as such, there is a strong cultural imperative to be with family members at the end of their lives. This often results in large numbers of GRT family members wanting to visit the hospital to pay their respects to the person who is dying whilst they are still alive. This is often in conflict with the wider cultural norms of smaller, nuclear families which influence hospital policies of limiting to one or two visitors at a time. Conversely, the example of breast feeding in maternity services where the cultural norm is bottle feeding and parents felt judged and '*… would either face stigma from within their community for choosing to breastfeed, or shame from health professionals if they chose to formula feed*' (FFT, 2024b; 5). These examples show a lack of understanding or respect for different cultural values held.

It is also important to note that most healthcare, particularly in the UK, is based upon the notion of equality, that is treating people the same. However, health inequity lies within social justice, recognising the unfair differences in health and health access are created due to structural and societal barriers. Therefore, to address health inequity, there needs to be an individualised approach, addressing the different barriers experienced by different groups. Put simply, there is nothing more unequal than the equal treatment of unequal people.

There is increasing recognition that there needs to be a shift in the education of health practitioners away from the traditional Eurocentric white male syllabus to include more women, Black and minority ethic, LGBT+ and disabled authors and content (Lokugamage et al., 2020). Within nursing and midwifery, there have been calls to decolonising pre and post registration educational programmes to address racialised and systematic inequities and to challenge the dominant discourses and ways of practicing (Thomas et al., 2025). This is often referred to as part of decolonising actions for curricula, which Bhambra et al. (2018) argue includes two main aspects: firstly, how ways of thinking about the world such as colonialism, empire and racism alongside other forms of discriminations have shaped the systems in which education is delivered and received; and secondly offering different ways of thinking and practising away from the status quo (Wong et al., 2021). Research by Marsh and Morgan (2025) exploring decolonising practices in 12 Universities in the UK identified that interviewees acknowledged they had not thought of including GRT in decolonising activities, despite recognising the importance of doing so. This missing inclusion reflects both institutional racism as well as the blind spot of 'white upon white' racism we discussed earlier. Furthermore, it ignores the colonisation of GRT who alike Indigenous Peoples have also experienced enforced cultural change (Heaslip et al., 2019a). We argue that any decolonising of nursing and midwifery curricula needs to include GRT to enable students to critically reflect on their values and beliefs to work in culturally sensitive ways (Heaslip et al., 2019b).

The Way Forward

Moving forwards, there needs to be the recognition that racism can and does occur in 'white against white' and that racism against minoritised communities, such as GRT, needs to have the same recognition and abhorrence as racism towards any other minoritised ethnic group. Thompson (2006) argues that oppression occurs at three distinct but interconnected levels (personal/psychological, cultural and structural), as such we argue that to address racism towards GRT then action also needs to occur at these levels.

Personal/Psychological

- Nurses and midwives need to explore their perceptions of GRT. To do this think of words that come to mind when you think of members of these communities, are they predominantly negative? In addition, when looking after GRT, do you automatically consider visiting in pairs, or are you anxious attending GRT sites? If this is so, develop an action plan to help you address your biases, this can include
  - Reading about GRT culture.
  - Critically reflecting on your perceptions, where do they stem from, is it actual experiences or through media reports and hearsay.
  - Read research conducted with these communities, do they offer a different perspective?
  - Challenging what you read in papers, it is factual or racialised bias.

- Nurse and midwives need to assess their understanding of GRT culture and examine whether they are practicing in culturally sensitive ways.
    - This can be achieved by linking to community groups, easily identified by searching the internet for GRT charities in your area. Reading their reports and accessing training programmes on GRT, Roma, Traveller culture. Success can be measured in an increased confidence and understanding of cultural values of these communities.
- Anti-Gypsyism should be openly discussed and labelled as racism. As a nurse or a midwife, do you challenge any anti-Gypsyism you encounter in your professional practice, if not, why? Success here would be measured by having a culture of no tolerance of racism or anti-Gypsyism.
- Nurses and midwives should assess whether their healthcare services meet the cultural needs of GRT. For example,
    - Linking to GRT community groups in the development of information, being mindful of literacy levels and using appropriate culturally sensitive language, as well as facilitating and respecting the informed choice of individuals.
    - Are there opportunities for women? GRT women to access someone of the same gender in appointments, particularly if discussing gynaecological, urinary or gastrointestinal issues.

Success here would be measured by asking GRT their experiences of accessing your services and whether they find your service culturally sensitive to their needs.

Cultural

- Research by the Equality and Human Rights Commission (2018) noted that GRT were perceived to be less deserving of equality and a lower priority in terms of seriousness of discrimination based on racialisation and ethnic minoritising. This must be addressed through the delivery of appropriate cultural safety training in all organisations, particularly health, education and policing.
- Anti-Gypsyism must be addressed through challenging inappropriate media representation and reporting any hate crime towards GRT to authorities. Furthermore, GRT communities must feel confident that reports of hate crime will be taken seriously by criminal justice services.

Structural

- The invisibilisation of GRT within data sets must be recognised as institutional racism. Data pertaining to these communities should be collated as a distinct subgroup within the white category, enabling a true understanding of their wider social determinants of health and health inequity.
- Nurses and midwives in primary care should undertake the Inclusion Health self-assessment tool available from https://www.inclusion-health.org/pcn/

Conclusion

This chapter has highlighted racism experienced by GRT at personal, cultural and structural levels both here in the UK and across Europe. It challenges the notion of racism being linked to skin colour alone, recognising the importance of both cultural and social status. It has highlighted the widespread anti-Gypsyism experienced by these communities and calls for it to be acknowledged as racism. Furthermore, it highlights the implications of racism on the lives of GRT and makes recommendations to ameliorate these.

Reflective Activity

Having read the chapter, we invite you to reflect on your key learning and its implications for your professional practice as a nurse or midwife using Bain et al.'s (2002) 5R framework (p. 13–15):

- Reporting – what is it in your situation you want to transform after reading this chapter?
- Responding – what are your personal observations regarding your own situation/context in relation to what is raised in this chapter?
- Relating – what is/are the theoretical/research/data/legislative, etc. understandings relationship to under consideration in this chapter that you could apply to your situation/context?
- Reasoning – Identify how the chapter findings matter to your situation/context and how will you interrogate your situation/context and what will help you from this chapter?
- Reconstructing – Identify your action plans to reframe and rebuild a transformative way forward to change from the situation in your context.

Notes

1. We use the term anti-Gypsyism as a collective term whilst recognising that not all Roma and Travellers identify as Gypsies.
2. This chapter does not focus on experiences of New Age Travellers, Boaters or Show people who are not perceived as minoritised ethnic.
3. It is important to recognise that Gypsy, Roma, Travellers are not the only 'white group' to experience racism, for example Jewish people have also historically and currently experience racism.

References

Abdalla, S., Kelleher, C.C., Quirke, B., and Daly, L.; on behalf of the All-Ireland traveller Health Study team. (2013). Disparities in Fatal and Nonfatal Injuries Between Irish Travellers and the Irish General Population Are Similar to Those of Other Indigenous Minorities: A Cross-Sectional Population-Based Comparative Study. *BMJ Open. 3*, e002296. https://doi.org/10.1136/bmjopen-2012-002296

Ahmed, S. (2006). *Queer Phenomenology*. Duke University Press.

Anastasaki, M., van Bree, E.M., Brakema, E.A., Tsiligianni, I., Sifaki-Pistolla, D., Chatzea, V.E., Crone, M.C., Karelis, A., van der Kleij, R.M.J.J., Poot, C.C., Reis, R., Chavannes, N.H., and Lionis, C. (2022). Beliefs, Perceptions, and Behaviors Regarding Chronic Respiratory Diseases of Roma in Crete, Greece: A Qualitative FRESH AIR Study. *Front Public Health. 15*(10), 812700. https://doi.org/10.3389/fpubh.2022.812700

Bain, J.D., Ballantyne, R., Mills, C., and Lester, N.C. (2002). *Reflecting on Practice: Student teachers' Perspectives*. Post Pressed.

Bhambra, G.K., Gebrial, D., and Nişancioğlu, K. (2018). *Decolonising the University*. Pluto Press.

Bhopal, K. and Myers, M. (2008). *Insiders, Outsiders and Others: Gypsies and Identity*. University of Hertfordshire Press.

Bloch, A. and Quarmby, K. (2024). Environmental Racism, Segregation and Discrimination: Gypsy and Traveller Sites in Great Britain. *Critical Social Policy, 45*(1), 94–114. https://doi.org/10.1177/02610183241229053

Borkowska, M., Nazroo, J., Finney, N., and Harrison, J., Ethnic identities (Chapter 3). In Finney, N., Nazroo, J., Bécares, L., Kapadia, D., Shlomo, N. (2023). *Racism and Ethnic Inequality in a Time of Crisis: Findings from the Evidence for Equality National Survey*. Policy Press.

Brown, P., Scullion, L., and Martin, P. (2013). *Migrant Roma in the United Kingdom: Population size and experiences of local authorities and partners*. https://pure.hud.ac.uk/en/publications/migrant-roma-in-the-united-kingdom-population-size-and-experience

Corradi, L. (2021). Intersectional Alliances to Overcome Gender Subordination: The Case of Roma-Gypsy Traveller Women. *Journal of International Women's Studies. 22*(4), 152–166.

Cunningham, C. and Stanley, F. (2003). Indigenous by definition, experience, or world view. *BMJ. 327*, 403. https://doi.org/10.1136/bmj.327.7412.403

Dagli, A. and Webb, R.T. (2025). Mental Illness and Suicidality Among Roma and Traveller Communities in the UK, Ireland, and Other Countries: A Systematic Review. *BMC Psychiatry. 25*(331). https://doi.org/10.1186/s12888-025-06752-0

Equality and Human Rights Commission. (2018). *Developing a national barometer of prejudice and discrimination in Britain*. https://www.equalityhumanrights.com/sites/default/files/national-barometer-of-prejudice-and-discrimination-in-britain.pdf

European Commission. (2020). *A Union of Equality: EU Roma strategic framework for equality, inclusion and participation*. https://commission.europa.eu/strategy-and-policy/policies/justice-and-fundamental-rights/combatting-discrimination/roma-eu/roma-equality-inclusion-and-participation-eu_en

European Union. (2019). *Discrimination in the European Union*. https://europa.eu/eurobarometer/surveys/detail/2251

European Union. (2023). *Discrimination in the European Union*. https://europa.eu/eurobarometer/surveys/detail/2972

European Union. (2024). *Report from the commission to the European parliament, the Council, the European Economic and Social Committee and the Committee of the Regions* https://eur-lex.europa.eu/legal-content/EN/TXT/PDF/?uri=COM:2024:422:FIN

European Union Agency for Fundamental Human Rights. (2020). *Roma and Travellers in six countries*. https://fra.europa.eu/en/publication/2020/roma-travellers-survey

European Union Agency for Fundamental Human Rights. (2021). *Roma in 10 European Countries*. https://fra.europa.eu/sites/default/files/fra_uploads/fra-2022-roma-survey-2021-main-results_en.pdf#page=51

Friends, Families and Travellers. (n.d.). *Nazi persecution and genocide of Roma and Sinti communities Introduction for teachers*. https://www.gypsy-traveller.org/wp-content/uploads/2025/03/Holocaust_Resource_Pack-2.pdf

Friends, Families and Travellers. (2022). *Briefing: Health inequalities experienced by Gypsy, Roma and Traveller communities*. https://www.gypsy-traveller.org/wp-content/uploads/2022/11/Briefing_Health-inequalities-experienced-by-Gypsies-and-Travellers-in-England.pdf

Friends, Families and Travellers. (2023). *Guidance: Tackling Maternal Health Inequalities in Gypsy, Roma and Traveller Communities.* https://www.gypsy-traveller.org/wp-content/uploads/2025/03/Extended-Maternal-Health-Inequalities-Guidance-2.pdf

Friends, Families and Travellers (2024a). High Court declares parts of Police Act 2022 in breach of European Convention on Human Rights. https://www.gypsy-traveller.org/campaign/high-court-declares-parts-of-police-act-2022-in-breach-of-european-convention-of-human-rights/#:~:text=Today%2C%20a%20High%20Court%20Judge,Act%201994%2C%20as%20incompatible%20with

Friends, Families and Travellers. (2024b). *Gypsy, Roma and Traveller community experiences of infant feeding, information and support services.* https://www.gypsy-traveller.org/wp-content/uploads/2024/09/Extended-Infant-Feeding-Report.pdf

Garner, S. (2017). Accommodation Crisis: the Racialization of Travellers in Twenty-First Century England. *Ethnic and Racial Studies. 42*(4), 511–530. https://doi.org/10.1080/01419870.2017.1380213

Gov.UK. (2025). *Count of Traveller Caravans, January 2025: England.* https://www.gov.uk/government/statistics/traveller-caravan-count-january-2025/count-of-traveller-caravans-january-2025-england#count-of-traveller-caravans

Greenfields, M. and Rogers, C. (2020). *Hate: "As regular as rain" a pilot research project into the psychological effects of hate crime on Gypsy, Traveller and Roma (GTR) communities.* https://gateherts.org.uk/wp-content/uploads/2020/12/Rain-Report-201211.pdf

Heaslip, V. (2015). *Experiences of Vulnerability from a Gypsy/Travelling Perspective: A Phenomenological Study, PhD.* Bournemouth University.

Heaslip, V., Hean, S., and Parker, J. (2016). Lived Experience of Vulnerability from a Gypsy Roma Traveller Perspective. *Journal of Clinical Nursing. 25*(13–4), 1987–1998.

Heaslip, V., Vanceulebroeck, V., Kalkan, I., Kömürcü, N., and Anton Solanas, I. (2019b). Student Nurse Perceptions of Gypsy Roma Travellers: A European Qualitative Study. *Nurse Education Today. 82*(Nov), 1–7. https://doi.org/10.1016/j.nedt.2019.07.011

Heaslip, V., Wilson, D., and Jackson, D. (2019a). Gypsy Roma Travellers: An Indigenous Population. *Public Health. 176*, 43–49. https://doi.org/10.1016/j.puhe.2019.02.020

Hutchison, P., Chihade, R., and Puiu, A.A. (2018). Predictors of "the Last Acceptable Racism": Group Threats and Public Attitudes Toward Gypsies and Travellers. *Journal of Applied Psychology. 48*(5), 237–247. https://doi.org/10.1111/jasp.12508

International Council of Nurses. (2021). *The ICN Code of Ethics for Nurses.* https://www.icn.ch/sites/default/files/inline-files/ICN_Code-of-Ethics_EN_Web.pdf

Irish Traveller Movement. (2019). *About Irish Travellers.* https://itmtrav.ie/what-is-itm/irish-travellers/

James, Z. (2021). Roma, Gypsies, and Travellers As a Community of Difference: Challenging Inclusivity as an Anti-racist Approach. *Critical Romani Studies. 4*(4), 142–162. https://doi.org/10.29098/crs.v4i2.104

Kirkby, A., Whitcombe, E., and Nuttall, E. (2023). *Briefing: Education inequalities facing Gypsies, Roma and Travellers in England, November 2023.* https://www.gypsy-traveller.org/wp-content/uploads/2025/03/Education-inequalities-faced-by-Gypsies-Roma-and-Travellers-in-England-briefing-2.pdf

Legislation.Gov.UK. (2026) Section 60C of the Criminal Justice and Public Order Act, 1994. https://www.legislation.gov.uk/ukpga/1994/33/section/60C

Legislation.gov.uk. (n.d). Equality Act 2010. https://www.legislation.gov.uk/ukpga/2010/15/contents

Lokugamage, A.U., Ahillan, T., and Pathberiya, S.D.C. (2020). Decolonising Ideas of Healing in Medical Education. *J Med Ethics. 46*, 265–272. https://doi.org/10.1136/medethics-2019-105866

Marsh, H. and Morgan, J. (2025). Decolonising the University Curriculum: An Investigation into Current Practice Regarding Gypsy, Roma and Traveller Communities. *Race Ethnicity and Education. 28*(6), 855–875. https://doi.org/10.1080/13613324.2025.2474936

McDonald, K.B. and Wingfield, A.M.H. (2008). (In)Visibility Blues: The Paradox of Institutional Racism. *Sociological Spectrum. 29*(1), 28–50. https://doi.org/10.1080/02732170802480501

NHS England. (2022). *Ethnicity*. https://digital.nhs.uk/data-and-information/data-collections-and-data-sets/data-sets/mental-health-services-data-set/submit-data/data-quality-of-protected-characteristics-and-other-vulnerable-groups/ethnicity

Nursing and Midwifery Council. (2018). *The Code*. https://www.nmc.org.uk/globalassets/sitedocuments/nmc-publications/nmc-code.pdf

O'Brien, M., Dempsey, B., and Higgins, M. (2024). The Experiences and Outcomes of Gypsy, Roma, and Traveller Pregnant People in Pregnancy: A Scoping Review. *Internal Journal of Gynaecology and Obstetrics. 167*(2), 529–537. https://doi.org/10.1002/ijgo.15723

Office for National Statistics. (2022a). *Gypsies' and Travellers' lived experiences, justice, England and Wales: 2022*. ttps://www.ons.gov.uk/peoplepopulationandcommunity/crimeandjustice/bulletins/gypsiesandtravellerslivedexperiencesjusticeenglandandwales/2022

Office for National Statistics. (2022b). *Gypsies' and Travellers' lived experiences, education and employment, England and Wales: 2022*. https://www.ons.gov.uk/peoplepopulationandcommunity/educationandchildcare/bulletins/gypsiesandtravellerslivedexperienceseducationandemploymentenglandandwales/2022

Office for National Statistics. (2022c). *Gypsies' and Travellers' lived experiences, health, England and Wales: 2022*. https://www.ons.gov.uk/peoplepopulationandcommunity/healthandsocialcare/healthcaresystem/bulletins/gypsiesandtravellerslivedexperienceshealthenglandandwales/2022

Rowlands, S., Heaslip, V., Felske-Durksen, C., Carranza Ko, N., Albert, G., Rich, R., Black, K.A., and Szilvási, M. (2024). The Forced Sterilisation of Indigenous and Racialised Peoples: Origins, Nature of Abuses, harms and Prevention. *International Perspectives on Health Equity*, 1750–6123. https://doi.org/10.1108/IPHEE-01-2024-0003

Ryden, J. (2013). Processes of oppression (Chapter 4). In V. Heaslip and J. Ryden (Ed.), *Understanding Vulnerability; a Nursing and Healthcare Approach* (pp. 65–90). Wiley.

Schwalbe, M., Godwin, S., Holden, D., Schrock, D., Thompson, S., and Wolkomir, M. (2000). Generic Processes in the Reproduction of Inequality: An Interactionist Analysis. *Social Forces. 79*(2), 419–452. https://doi.org/10.1093/sf/79.2.419

Sierra, M. (2024). *The Roma and the Holocaust*. Bloomsbury Publishing.

Stephan, W.G., Ybarra, O., and Morrison, K.R. (2009). Intergroup threat theory. In T.D. Nelson (Ed.), *Handbook of Prejudice, Stereotyping, and Discrimination* (pp. 43–59). Psychology Press.

Thomas, S., Allan, G., Heaslip, V., and Furber, C. (2025). A Systematic Review of Key Principles Relating to Decolonising Interventions in Midwifery Education. *Women and Birth. 38*(2). https://doi.org/10.1016/j.wombi.2025.101869

Thompson, N. (2006). *Anti-Discriminatory Practice*, 4th Edition. Palgrave Macmillan.

Thompson, N. (2011). *Promoting Equality: Working With Diversity and Difference*, 3rd Edition. Palgrave Macmillan.

Thompson, N. and Woodger, D. (2020). "I hope the river Floods": Online Hate Speech Towards Gypsy, Roma and Traveller Communities. *British Journal of Community Justice. 16*(1), 41–63.

Traveller Movement. (2017). *The last acceptable form of racism? The pervasive discrimination and prejudice experienced by Gypsy, Roma and Traveller communities*. https://travellermovement.org.uk/policy-and-publications/the-last-acceptable-form-of-racism

Traveller Movement. (2022). *Number of Gypsy, Roma, and Traveller people disclosing ethnicity in census increases by 110,000*. https://travellermovement.org.uk/news/5719

Tremlett, A. (2023). Challenging Stereotypes Is Not Enough: A Dialogue With Roma Art. *Journal of Cultural Analysis and Social Change. 8*(2), 09. https://doi.org/10.20897/jcasc/14062

UK Parliament. (2024). *Gypsies, Roma and Travellers: Statistics*. https://commonslibrary.parliament.uk/research-briefings/cbp-10063/

Wilson, D., Heaslip, V., and Jackson, D. (2018). Improving Equity and Cultural Responsiveness With Marginalised Communities: Understanding Competing Worldviews. *Journal of Clinical Nursing*. *27*(19–20), 3810–3819. https://doi.org/10.1111/jocn.14546

Wong, S.H.M., Gishen, F., and Lokugamage, A.U. (2021). "Decolonising the Medical Curriculum": Humanising Medicine Through Epistemic Pluralism, Cultural Safety and Critical Consciousness. *London Review of Education*, *19*(1), 1–22. https://doi.org/10.14324/LRE.19.1.16

World Health Organization. (2021). *Building better together roadmap to guide implementation of the global strategic directions for nursing and midwifery in the WHO European region*. https://www.who.int/europe/publications/i/item/WHO-EURO-2021-4464-44227-62471

12

ANTI-RACISM HEALING

Timothea T. Vo

Introduction

The purpose of this chapter is to introduce the idea of radical healing for all nurse providers – nurse educators, nurse scientists, nurse midwives, nurse practitioners, nurse historians, nurse executives, among other healthcare professionals who have invested in doing anti-racism work.

Anti-racism healing is emphasizing that anti-racism work is systemic, multiple points of actions to lead to diminishing individual health harms, amending disparities, reducing detrimental racialized discriminations, and cultivating relational robustness. This will bring together people and communities regardless of their racialization to heal together as a social movement for radical anti-racism change work (Integrity Coaching, 2025). The cumulative negative effects of racism on the human psyche are most consequential. According to the National Commission to Address Racism in Nursing (2021), being a recipient of interpersonal racism/microaggression is equivalent to an assault on the human mind, body, and spirit. When one's energy, time, and resources are usurped to process experiences of everyday racism, it causes lasting harm to one's physical and mental health, leading to feelings of worthlessness (Williams *et al.*, 1997). As a result of this, racialized persons experience higher levels of anxiety, depression, chronic stress, low self-esteem, loneliness, anger, and suicidality (Mind UK, 2021). Racism, discriminations, oppressions, and injustices are experienced by every person doing the anti-racism work, but paradoxically doing the work is healing, changing, and transformative because the work is relational. Although this chapter is primarily from the US context, the content is globally transferable.

Healing is a form of resistance to the status quo.

DOI: 10.4324/9781003565369-12

It is not uncommon for nurse providers and midwives of color who are committed to root out racism as a whole in clinical practice and/or academic settings to also experience re-traumatization (Esaki *et al.*, 2022). This is because anti-racism work continually raises and revisits, reminds and reawakens the harms, oppressions, and injustices experienced in their lifetimes due to racism (American Psychological Association, 2021). It is crucial, if not vital, to honor the healing it takes to move forward with equity and justice focused action for nursing and midwifery healthcare. To continue doing anti-racism work well, nurses and midwives must remain attentive to also doing the things which give them joy in this shared journey to let heal what hurts us all (Everybody's Work, 2023), lest the emotional, physical, and spiritual toll of anti-racism justice activism leads to burnout in the already stressful disciplines of nursing and midwifery (Gorski and Erakat, 2019). Joy is also resistance to the status quo. Hence, we must acknowledge the courage and moral fortitude it takes to continue engaging in anti-racism work in different spaces and places. Therefore, this chapter serves to provide ways for all nurses and midwives at every level of practice or leadership to engage in anti-racism healing, a way to disrupt racism in the healthcare system.

Anti-Racism Healing – A Six Components Framework

While racism has been a long-standing issue in society, studies show nurse providers have also experienced racism in healthcare (Walsh *et al.*, 2025). In 2022, researchers at the University of Chicago conducted a study of 980 nurses to examine the prevalence and impact of racism and discrimination in the workplace and nursing schools in the United States (Robert Wood Johnson Foundation, 2023). Findings demonstrated that most Black/African American and Asian nurses have seen or experienced racism or discrimination from both patients and colleagues, supporting the fact that racism is pervasive in nursing. Of the sample, 88 percent of Black nurses experienced racist actions and behaviors from patients, and 72 percent reported experiencing racism or discrimination from colleagues (Robert Wood Johnson Foundation, 2023). Asian nurses reported similar responses, noting microaggressive behavior in the form of racial slurs (e.g., comments like "Tramp stamps" or "Where are you really from?") from patients and even their coworkers. Unfortunately, these incidents of racism and discrimination were ubiquitous for nurses of color, and portrayed by patients (79%) more frequently than workplace colleagues (59%) (Robert Wood Johnson Foundation, 2023). According to anti-racist birth equity researcher, Dr. Monica McLemore, "Nursing and social justice have been mutually aligned since the inception of nursing" (@shiftnursing, 2024).

As justice takes on different forms, so does healing. The following discussions will be separated using an adapted version of the six components subheadings for anti-racist healing originally created by Integrity Coaching (2025), that is:

(a) Understanding Self to Heal

Racial inequities of stress are pronounced, and white nurses have consistently avoided talking about racism in the name of *white fragility* (McIntosh, 2003; DiAngelo, 2018). Moreover, white nurses' refusal(s) to step up when called upon, uphold the established idea of hierarchical white/Black racialized structures in nursing, akin to the unjust segregation seen during the Civil Rights era (Iheduru-Anderson, 2021). This inaction or hesitation in times where humanity has been deeply violated and wronged shows that silence is not always golden but rather complicit in violence, whether that be spiritual, mental, or physical (Library of Congress, 2021). In the disappointment of this quietude, the trumpet voice of Dr. Reverend Martin Luther King, Jr. emblazons on the collective conscience, *"In the end, we will remember not the words of our enemies, but the silence of our friends"* (King, 1968, p. 78). When *whiteness* has been a historically favored focal point, nursing faculty and students of color are negatively impacted, and may be forced to look, act or speak in manners like them, which can lead to cultural alienation and further silence from certain groups (Vo, 2021). Therefore, authentic allyship and active listening from white nurses and midwives are needed to actively speak up (be loud) and speak out (be in the conversation) about injustice while joining in the work of change, to start the healing process of justice for all in the anti-racism work.

Anti-racism service to the field takes a significant toll on the mind, body, and spirit and can result in burnout (Gorski and Erakat, 2019) across all racialized bodies. Despite this, most nurses of color recognized their moral imperative to address racism in different forms. Therefore, anti-racism work is often tasked by women of color (e.g., Black, Hispanic, Latina, Asian, Indigenous) and/or from historically and socially marginalized communities (Danquah *et al.*, 2021). This frank reminder encourages *all* nurses to enter self-reflection as accountable and responsible patient advocates, and/or anti-racism activists, to help disrupt and eventually dismantle racism. Anti-racism disruption leads to safety for receivers and deliverers of healthcare. Reflection is used as a tool to identify internal bias/es, to unlearn racism, to expose internal oppressions and relearn to be and do radically differently to contribute to systemic anti-racism change making. This is healing because it helps to understand what is enjoyable, what is challenging, hence when to rest, what and who to avoid to keep going.

For nurses doing the anti-racism work, to heal there is opportunity to apply a heart-centered approach (RICHER Model). Using music and movement can help nurses and midwives process stress, reconnect with joy, and promote well-being to reclaim their inner freedom (Nwankpa, 2025). As burnout and stress continue to increase in nursing – healing is crucial, if not vital when doing the anti-racism work – and must be done with *intentionality*. Through embodied, creative, and culturally-oriented approaches, nurses and midwives can engage in their own anti-racist healing process and slowly integrate their mind, body, and spirit connectivity

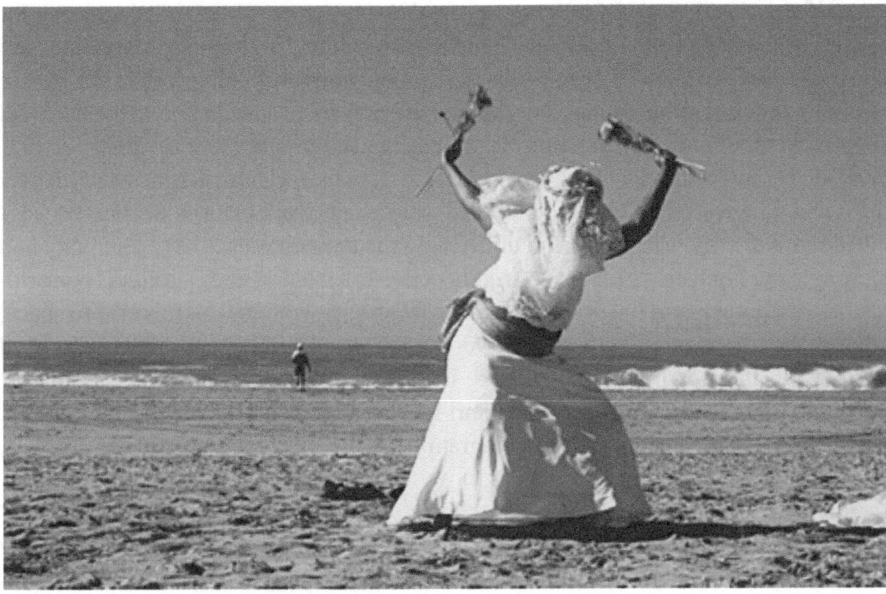

FIGURE 12.1 RICHER Model: Re-indigenizing wellness through evidence-based healing arts (Nwankpa, 2025)

Sources: Picture used with permission of creator Dr. Uzo Nwankpa.

themselves. This includes, but is not limited to expressive arts healing, such as music, meditation, traditional or contemporary dance that leaves one with a type of relaxation, calmness, reenergizing and regeneration that satisfies and brings joy (Figure 12.1).

The black and white picture is of a person performing a ritual dance on Ocean Beach, CA. The central figure is wearing a short sleeved full-length wide-skirt white dress outfit, with a darker bandana tied around their hips. They wear a white lacy head scarf the length at the back is to their waist and it is held onto their head with a flower bandeau. In their hands they hold slim bouquet of flowers. They have a wide leg stance, body slightly forward, and knees bent. The upper part of their body is fully twisted, so that only their back is visible and their arms are raised above their heads.

Expressive arts healing commences by taking each letter of the acronym, RICHER, *R stands for Self Reflection; I – Integration (mind, body, and spirit); CH – Choreography (breathe, move, shake); E – Evaluation (objective assessment); R – Self-Reflection* again, and engaging with it for as much/as long as one needs, or is able. Results may vary.

For people to sustain themselves in the long haul work of anti-racism, they must do self-care. Audre Lorde (1988, p. 130), a civil rights activist, poet, and writer, said of self-care that it is a radical act and that, *"Caring for myself is not self-indulgence, it is self-preservation, and that is an act of political warfare."* Meaning that caring for oneself is in itself a form of resistance to the harms of racism trauma, oppression, and injustices. She promoted that self-care was not only about keeping well in the face of adversity but also maintaining your dignity and powers to sustain you in the hard and lengthy work of anti-racism. Anti-racism change starts with the individual persons' themselves, understanding their positions and actions for anti-racism, what hinders them and what can they pull on to do the anti-racism work. This is healing because the individual starts to explore and understand the resources they have internally and their agency. Nguyen (2025), civil rights activist, sexual assault survivor, bioastronautics researcher, and the first Vietnamese American woman who traveled to space, advises that those doing anti-racism work, such as in nursing and midwifery, need to invest in their own healing, because justice takes on different forms. Being involved in your wellbeing while doing anti-racism work is part of that healing justice. Nguyen (2025) further says in an Instagram post:

> *It is admirable to want to help the world. And if that life of justice calls you, I will be there to fight alongside you. But I also want you to know it's ok– it's ok if you only save one person. And it's ok it that person is you. Joy is the most radical form of rebellion. My wish for all is that you can find that healing, justice, and joy.*

(b) Closing/reducing Group Disparities

Lots of actions are taken to reduce the differences between groups regarding healthcare experiences. This is healing the communities and oneself if you belong to a group that is in receipt of inequitable services. Blatant racial injustice from birth was clearly unacceptable, and spurred nurses and midwives to advocate for specific educational health reforms. Specifically, Black midwives broke through the mold by building midwifery schools that accepted and enrolled Black students into midwifery schools and colleges, who trained and learned how to become midwives, graduating from their midwifery program to essentially provide direct, life-saving care for marginalized Black mothers and babies, families, and communities (Canty, 2025; Olden and Yada, 2025). According to Mitchell-Miland *et al.* (2023), inclusive mentorship experiences from senior or mid-career doctorate nurses of color will aid in the advancement of nurses who are navigating nursing school or academia for the first time (e.g., first nurse in their family, doctoral student, doctorly prepared nurse practitioner or researcher). By sharing and investing in their postgraduate professional experiences, early career nurse scholars and nurse scientists can better research innovative approaches, produce award-winning publications, and grants to understand cultural health, explore uncharted phenomena, implement tried-and-true health interventions to reduce health disparities in their community of research.

There is healing from knowledge generation and dissemination. Nursing and midwifery research is an important area where researchers have an opportunity to exercise epistemic justice by citing high-quality, peer-reviewed publications of researchers of color who are addressing systemic and structural racism. Smith *et al.* (2021) disseminated a hashtag #CiteBlackWomen via the Cite Black Women Collective @ (http://www.citeblackwomencollective.org/) to elevate, spotlight, and encourage the publications of Black women stemming from different professions, sectors, and fields. For example, citing Black women is essential to any discipline as it advances and contributes to the growing body of literature. According to Cayo (2025), this not only addresses patriarchal and historical roots of hegemony and racism, but directly credits both individual and collective knowledge to Black women that white men and then white women in science had monopolized exclusively. Black maternal health scholars in the community raised public awareness about the US maternal health crisis affecting Black women, who are two to three times more likely to die during childbirth compared to white women (McLemore and D'Efilippo, 2019; Scott *et al.*, 2019). These large data helped inform legislation to address Black maternal morbidity and mortality as a public health issue. Healing can be through delivering justice by disrupting the dominance of white researchers in the field of Black healthcare.

Nurses from all over the world were called to become anti-racist in different spaces and places at the patients' bedsides, classrooms and boardrooms, clinics and homes (Bennett *et al.*, 2019; Koschmann *et al.*, 2020). For example, nurse educators sought to dismantle racism in nursing by revising curriculum and defining health equity for the new millennia (Lewis *et al.*, 2023; Waite *et al.*, 2024). Nurses and midwives became voices of change, doubling down on principles and values of trauma-informed care to protect and foster a truly anti-racist culture (Esaki *et al.*, 2022; The National Commission to Address Racism in Nursing, 2021). In this shared effort to dismantle racism in healthcare, organizations such as the American Association of Colleges of Nursing (AACN) and National League for Nursing (NLN) strongly spoke out against racism in nursing education (AACN, 2024). The AACN and NLN jointly stated, "We stand together against attacks to censor and dismantle programs that educate students and nursing providers about all forms of racism and promote inclusion" (AACN, 2024). This includes acknowledging that racism exists in the healthcare system. These statements were faced with support and resistance as it would possibly disrupt structures or dismantle systems irrevocably changing them, from functioning with an unchecked, *lawless* spirit of racism as traditional.

Research doings, knowledge sharing, and education applying anti-racism approach will heal communities, because it is focused on reducing disparities that harm, oppress, and create inequity in life and health experiences and journeys.

(c) Intentional Interconnectedness

Historically, nurses have been in a perfect position to link arms in the name of social justice, caring, and healing, especially during times of civil and societal unrest

(Abu, 2020). For example, during the Civil Rights Movement (1950s–1970s), significant momentum was achieved when *both* white and Black/African American nurses actively opposed racism. Claire O'Connor, a white nurse, demonstrably stood in the segregated "colored" restroom and got arrested, and Josephine "Jo" Disparti, another white nurse delivered life-saving medical care in the middle of the night to wounded African American pregnant women, who otherwise would not receive proper care under Jim Crow laws (Pollitt, 2016). Rachel Robinson, wife to major league baseball player, Jackie Robinson, decried the injustice of blatant systemic racism while Black people in her community and other persons of color residing in low-income neighborhoods were dying under the oppressive forces (Pollitt, 2016). These were set forth by the racial segregation system which denied them access to prominent healthcare facilities where white patients had stayed (Pollitt, 2016). Members of online communities who wrote freely about social justice via different social media platforms uplifted people with words of encouragement and support. These posts affirmed peoples' lived experiences of racism and identified allies in the anti-racist movement as well (Brannon, 2023). Joy is healing and resistance to the status quo.

There is healing in working together as a group. This was established by Yalom (1970) in his identification of 11 curative factors for group work that enable individual change through being in a group with purpose. In this chapter, these are explained in terms of their relation to anti-racism healing:

1 Instillation of hope – Doing the work and seeing progression gives rise to believing there is a way forward to change racism in the system.
2 Universality – Knowing you are not alone and there are others who share your problems and who are doing the anti-racism change work.
3 Imparting information – There is a sharing of stories and knowledge that support and strengthen the group in their work.
4 Altruism – Helping others can be a healing experience, as it is related to 1, 2, and 3.
5 Corrective Recapitulation of the Primary Family Group – Re-experiencing positive family type dynamics in a nurturing safe space, this can create belonging when feeling isolated doing the anti-racism work/activism.
6 Development of Socializing Techniques – Gaining confidence in articulating your vision, mission, and values in doing the anti-racism work creates better connections with the group.
7 Imitative Behavior – Learning from others in the group to improve how you do your anti-racism work so you don't burn out.
8 Interpersonal Learning – Learning about yourself in this work and how to do the work better with every interaction within the group.
9 Group Cohesiveness – Feeling belonging, knowing you are not alone, and feeling psychological safety within a group doing the anti-racism work.

10 Catharsis – Storytelling can help reduce stress and improve emotional wellbeing. With storytelling anti-racist nurses and midwives can unveil opportunities for growth and (self) healing as their light can shine through those "fractured" places of their mind, body, and soul addressing barriers and strategies for sustainable anti-racism progress (Houskova *et al.*, 2024).
11 Existential Factors – Knowing you are free to be responsible, even if it leads to necessary disruptive activities for the greater good.

However, researchers have warned about the challenges of collective action efforts, as they become more powerful and gain momentum with large-scale success, where strong attempts to silence activists will likely occur simultaneously (Matthews and Zukowska, 2025). Therefore, anti-racist nurses and midwives must aim to guard themselves against the critics and *noise* that are external to this inherent *life-or-death* health justice issue. Nursing and midwifery leadership invested in anti-racism and models of collective action can help provide clear guidance and direction to members of their professional organizations to determine ways anti-racism can sustain power and impact beyond its movement.

(d) Transformation

Today, healthcare inequities are based in long-standing systemic racism, contributing to poor (yet preventable) intergenerational health outcomes. Unequal treatment based on race alone is considered a manufactured social construct perpetuated by other people wanting to hold on to their power and privilege (Gannon, 2016). Anti-racist leadership developed think tanks to protect and redefine the future of the disciplines. For example, in 2021, the National Commission to Address Racism in Nursing focusing on (re)writing, adjusting, and amplifying language and initiatives that center on first: understanding racism, introducing new definitions, and promoting anti-racism praxis that all nurses can adopt. According to the National Commission to Address Racism in Nursing (2021), on the American Association of Nursing website, racism was reviewed by a commission of panel of experts and redefined as:

> *Assaults on the human spirit in the form of actions, biases, prejudices, and an ideology of superiority based on race that persistently cause moral suffering and physical harm of individuals and perpetuate systemic injustices and inequities*
>
> *(National Commission to Address Racism in Nursing, 2021)*

Anti-racism organization transformation is healing because it shifts minds and behaviors to do the just thing and deliver equitable nursing and midwifery healthcare, fostering belonging through psychological safety. The latter term means that individuals within teams in organizations can be open about discussing racism and discriminations without fear of reprisal (Edmondson, 2019). This leads to more motivated teams, better decision-making, and a culture of continuous improvement because people feel belonging (McKinsey and Company, 2023). McKinsey and Company's (2015, p. 1) study identified that these mind shifts and behavioral change in people in organizations happen due to four critical key factors: "role modeling, fostering understanding and conviction, reinforcing changes through formal mechanisms, and developing talent and skills." Everyone involved in or moving toward anti-racism work, including in nursing and midwifery, will be embedding themselves within these factors and committed anti-racism leadership will design effective initiatives for the successful outcomes from the four factors. This is a healthy embodied nourishing and healing in the workplace environment.

Furthermore, the transformation of self is continuously happening in the anti-racism work and space due to a, b, c, and d. Individual healing is influenced by the internal and external environment, as are groups/teams and organizations. Lean into healing from anti-racism change and see how you transform on a personal, family, and work level, because we learn and develop through change and interactions in contexts.

(e) Building Anti-Racism Futures

In times where it was wildly unpopular to speak up for communities of color, who today are still oppressed, marginalized, and often silenced, communities of color rely on anti-racist nurses and midwives to continue championing spaces and places with equity-minded action that informs culturally-concordant theory and practice (Solomon *et al.*, 2019). There is too much at stake, as opportunities abound to make a difference in the lives of the communities anti-racist nurses and midwives continue helping and serving. For example, the ethical and honest attributes inherent within the nursing profession manifest in ways that not only facilitate life-saving care, but also treatment approaches that encompass the holistic art, science, and ways of knowing (Brown *et al.*, 2022). Nurses have the natural instinct to meet people in the moment through empathy and respect shown with hearts of compassion and hands of healing. Therefore, nurses are in the perfect position to confront racism as a true public health crisis due to the nature of being on the frontlines where nursing care and possibilities of patient healing collide.

What's more, engaging in anti-racist justice activism reflects the ethos of the nursing and midwifery professions which emphasizes empathy, caring, and social justice. Historically, nursing has been referred to as a calling, yet nursing is also a profession that requires years of rigorous training, accountability, responsibility, highly skilled labor, and safe practice. For 23 consecutive years, Gallup's Honesty and Ethics of Professions Poll reported that most Americans (three out of four) have named nursing as the number one trusted profession (Saad, 2025). According to the American Nurses Association (2025), the updated Code of Ethics places a stronger emphasis on upholding human dignity, patient rights and autonomy; promoting global health communities; engaging in self-care and nurse well-being; and eradicating systemic and structural racism (American Nurses Association, 2025). These provisions reflect what was declared in Paris, France, on December 10, 1948 by the United Nations General Assembly Resolution 217 A that the principles of equal treatment and non-discrimination based on "race, colour, sex, language, religion, political or other opinion, national or social origin, property, birth or other status" are cornerstones of one's human rights (United Nations, 1948, 2021).

The *Future of Nursing 2020–2030* report underscores that diversifying the workforce and continuing nursing professional development are key areas for strengthening the nursing profession over time (Wakefield *et al.*, 2021). In 2022, shared efforts between AACN and funding from Johnson & Johnson sought to better support retention and diversity in the workforce by implementing digital tools to identify practices that promote belongingness among underrepresented nursing students and faculty (American Association of Colleges of Nursing, 2023). Support and promotion of nurses from historically social and marginalized groups in all substantive healthcare settings and undergraduate and graduate nursing pathways are needed. By harnessing the talents and skills of a diverse nurse workforce, better health outcomes and healthy communities can be realized (Bradford *et al.*, 2022, 2025).

(f) Re-imagining and Rebuilding an Anti-Racism Profession

Nurses and midwives have the gumption, moral courage, and passion to care for people in their greatest time of need. By leading with compassionate care and skill, the human condition and integrity of the profession are maintained. As our commitment and unwavering drive to health equity persists, we also need to let the flow of healing enter our bodies, minds, and hearts, lest the physical, mental, and emotional toll of anti-racist work leads to burnout in an already stressful discipline. Nurses and midwives new to anti-racist justice activism are welcome to enter the movement at any time. Being anti-racist does not have to be forced or embellished with banners or picket signs. Patient advocacy can begin at the bedside, within communities, through transnational partnerships, across hiring practices, in research, theory development, and back to practice. Blatant acts of racism and discrimination in modern society have challenged people's gumption, insomuch that giving up is not an option on the table because lives and those whom nurses and midwives care about depend on it.

As nursing and midwifery professionals look to advance racial equity and meet this moment with open minds and an unquenchable thirst to dismantle structural racism in their institutions, organizations, and health systems, an *enlarging of the tent* initiative is crucial if we are to work together across organizational hierarchies to drive systemic change, especially during times of sociopolitical uncertainty (Robert Wood Johnson Foundation, 2025). For years before Diversity, Equity, and Inclusion (DEI) initiatives were developed, nurses from organizations such as Black Nurses Association, National Association of Hispanic Nurses, and the American Nurses Association have been thought leaders and champions condemning racism in nursing (Beard and Fields, 2025). Nurse leaders have precisely desired sustainable change for anti-racism in nursing. Banded together, these nursing organizations have aligned, instilling a broad sense of justice, equity, diversity, and belonging (JEDI) to hundreds of thousands of members and their proud associates. Anti-racist nurses have one thing in common, gumption. They say what they mean, and mean what they say. They lead with compassionate advocacy, speak with conviction, and act with moral fortitude to continue embodying equity-minded theory and practice.

Conclusion

Today, there are approximately five million nurses in the United States. From the genesis of nursing, nurses are called to lead with advocacy, integrity, and moral responsibility even in the face of adversity. Ethics are essential and the backbone of our profession – guiding every healing touch, assessment, and care provision. Nursing and midwifery go hand-in-hand with social justice. The social interconnectedness of our very discipline with patients, families, and the communities we serve stems from being a trustworthy source of information and knowledge to provide care for the minoritized and most marginalized. However, equity in anti-racism action is needed as racism continues to be a public health crisis. The times we are living in justify our needs and our call for anti-racism praxis. By doing this shared work together, we are not siloed, but rather a coalition of activists committed to eradicate racism. In the words of Dr. Ibram Kendi:

> *[We must] believe in the possibility that we can strive to be anti-racist from this day forward. Believe in the possibility that we can transform our societies to be anti-racist from this day forward. Racist power is not godly. Racist policies are not indestructible. Racial inequities are not inevitable. Racist ideas are not natural to the human mind.*
>
> *(cited in website American Association of Colleges of Nursing, 2024)*

As long as anti-racism activism efforts continue, anti-racism healing will become all the more urgent. Nurses and midwives need to embrace *and* empower each other through self-care and collaborative efforts. Therefore, we need to get to know each other better across organizational hierarchies, and especially hearing and knowing what other members are saying and doing, such as similar projects, research, or creative activities that address racism in healthcare. In this new millennium, each of us, as nurses and midwives of color, is beckoned by those who have gone before us, to come out from the shadows of silence. It is time to heal, raise our voices, and speak boldly with great clarity of our vision for a new world. We must and can choose to face this third millennium with emboldened vision, hopes, and dreams of the highest caliber. The choice is ours.

Reflective Activity

You are invited to reflect on the chapter and relate to your context using Bain *et al.*'s (2002) 5R framework (pp. 13–15):

- Reporting – what is it in your situation you want to transform after reading this chapter?
- Responding – what are your personal observations regarding your own situation/context in relation to what is raised in this chapter?
- Relating – what is/are the theoretical/research/data/legislative, etc. understandings relationship to under consideration in this chapter that you could apply to your situation/context?
- Reasoning – Identify how the chapter findings matter to your situation/context and how will you interrogate your situation/context and what will help you from this chapter?
- Reconstructing – Identify your action plans to reframe and rebuild a transformative way forward to change from the situation in your context.

References

@shiftnursing. (2024). *Nursing and social justice have been mutually aligned since the inception of nursing.* [Instagram]. 27 March. [Accessed 29 March 2024]. https://www.instagram.com/shiftnursing/p/C5BSpC6Mrei/?hl=am-et

Abu, V.K. (2020). Let us be unequivocal about social justice in nursing. *Nurse Education in Practice*, *47*, 102849. doi: 10.1016/j.nepr.2020.102849.

American Association of Colleges of Nursing. (2023). *Enhancing diversity in the nursing workforce*. https://www.aacnnursing.org/news-data/fact-sheets/enhancing-diversity-in-the-nursing-workforce

American Association of Colleges of Nursing. (2024). *Combatting racism in nursing education.* https://www.aacnnursing.org/news-data/all-news/combatting-racism-in-nursing-education

American Nurses Association. (2025). *2025 Code of Ethics provisions*. https://codeofethics.ana.org/provisions

American Psychological Association. (2021). *Managing your distress in the aftermath of racial trauma and stress.* https://www.apa.org/topics/racism-bias-discrimination/managing-distress-racial-trauma

Bain, J.D., Ballantyne, R., Mills, C. and Lester, N.C. (2002). *Reflecting on practice: Students teachers' perspectives*. Post Pressed.

Beard, K. and Fields, S. (2025). The genesis of the academy of diversity leaders in nursing. *American Journal of Nursing*, *125*(2), 16–17. doi: 10.1097/AJN.0000000000000012.

Bennett, C., Hamilton, E.K. and Rochani, H. (2019). Exploring race in nursing: Teaching nursing students about racial inequality using the historical Lens. *Online Journal of Issues in Nursing*, *24*(2). doi: 10.3912/OJIN.Vol24No02PPT20

Bradford, H.M., Bradley, P.K., Gomes, M., Simpson, K.R., Tilden, E.L., Lyndon, A., Krulewitch, C., Alexander, I.M. and Trego, L.L. (2025). Growth and diversification of the perinatal Nursing workforce: An American Academy of Nursing consensus paper. *Nursing Outlook, 73*(3), 102393. doi: 10.1016/j.outlook.2025.102393

Bradford, H.M., Grady, K., Kennedy, M.B. and Johnson, R.L. (2022). Advancing faculty diversity in nursing education: Strategies for success. *Journal of Professional Nursing, 42*, 239–249. doi: 10.1016/j.profnurs.2022.07.006.

Brannon, T.N. (2023). Racism hurts, can anti-racism heal?: Positive mental health correlates of anti-racist engagement. *Proceedings of the National Academies of Sciences Nexus, 2*(10), pgad309. doi: 10.1093/pnasnexus/pgad309.

Brown, B., Dillard-Wright, J., Hopkins-Walsh, J., Littzen, C.O.R. and Vo, T. (2022). Patterns of knowing and being in the COVIDicene: An epistemological and ontological reckoning for posthumans. *Advances in Nursing Science, 45*(1), 3–21. doi: 10.1097/ANS.0000000000000387.

Canty, L. (2025). Historical study of the graduates of the Tuskegee School of Nurse-Midwifery, a program for Black Nurses. *Journal of Obstetric, Gynecologic, and Neonatal Nursing, 54*(3), 349–360.e5. doi: 10.1016/j.jogn.2024.08.002.

Cayo, S. (2025). Advancing anti-racism. *American Nurse Journal, 20*(1). doi: 10.51256/ANJ012551.

Danquah, R., Lopez, C., Wade, L. and Castillo, L.G. (2021). Racial justice activist burnout of women of color in the United States: Practical tools for counselor intervention. *International Journal for the Advancement of Counseling, 43*(4), 519–533. doi: 10.1007/s10447-021-09449-7.

DiAngelo, R. (2018). *White fragility: Why it's so hard for white people to talk about racism.* Beacon Press.

Edmondson, A.C. (2019). *The fearless organization: Creating psychological safety in the workplace for learning, innovation, and growth.* John Wiley & Sons, Inc.

Esaki, N., Reddy, M. and Bishop, C.T. (2022). Next steps: Applying a trauma-informed model to create an anti-racist organizational culture. *Behavioral Sciences (Basel, Switzerland), 12*(2), 41. doi: 10.3390/bs12020041.

Everybody's Work. (2023). [YouTube]. *Directed by Chad Tingle. United States: Robert Wood Johnson Foundation and SHIFT Nursing.* https://www.youtube.com/watch?v=Qzmw3RBN_QA&list=PL8At-TNTcj0ys-u9Ya1R4do08ILrrrXA5&index=24

Gannon, M. (2016). *Race is a social construct, scientists argue*. Scientific American. https://www.scientificamerican.com/article/race-is-a-social-construct-scientists-argue/

Gorski, P.C. and Erakat, N. (2019). Racism, whiteness, and burnout in anti-racism movements: How white racial justice activists elevate burnout in racial justice activists of color in the United States. *Ethnicities, 19*(5), 784–808. doi: 10.1177/1468796819833871.

Houskova, M., Todd, C. and King, A. (2024). Anti-racism in nursing. *American Nurse Journal, 19*(11). doi: 10.51256/ANJ112423.

Iheduru-Anderson, K.C. (2021). The White/Black hierarchy institutionalizes White supremacy in nursing and nursing leadership in the United States. *Journal of Professional Nursing, 37*(2), 411–421. doi: 10.1016/j.profnurs.2020.05.005.

Integrity Coaching. (2025). *Anti-racist work: Bridging divides and cultivating wholeness.* https://www.integritycoaching.co.uk/blog/race-equality-and-diversity/anti-racist-work-healing-and-unity/

King, M.L. (1968). *The trumpet of conscience*. Beacon Press.

Koschmann, K.S., Jeffers, N.K. and Heidari, O. (2020). 'I can't breathe': A call for anti-racist nursing practice. *Nursing Outlook, 68*(5), 539–541. doi: 10.1016/j.outlook.2020.07.004.

Lewis, C.L., Yan, A., Williams, M.Y., Apen, L.V., Crawford, C.L., Morse, L., Valdez, A.M., Alexander, G.R., Grant, E., Valderama-Wallace, C. and Beatty, D. (2023). Health equity: A concept analysis. *Nursing Outlook, 71*(5), 102032. doi: 10.1016/j.outlook.2023.102032.

Library of Congress (2021). *White silence is violence – Black Lives Matter*. https://www.loc.gov/item/2022632922/

Lorde. A. (1988). *A burst of light: And other essays.* Courier Dover Publications.
Matthews, S. and Zukowska, M. (2025). *Liberation stories: Building narrative power for 21st century social movements.* New Press.
McIntosh, P. (2003). White privilege: Unpacking the invisible knapsack. In Plous, S. (ed.), *Understanding prejudice and discrimination.* McGraw-Hill, pp. 191–196.
McKinsey and Company. (2015). *The science of organisational transformations.* https://www.mckinsey.com/capabilities/people-and-organizational-performance/our-insights/the-science-of-organizational-transformations#/
McKinsey and Company. (2023). *Diversity matters even more: The case for holistic impact.* https://www.mckinsey.com/featured-insights/diversity-and-inclusion/diversity-matters-even-more-the-case-for-holistic-impact#/
McLemore, M. and D'Efilippo, V. (2019). *To prevent women from dying in childbirth, first stop blaming them.* https://www.scientificamerican.com/article/to-prevent-women-from-dying-in-childbirth-first-stop-blaming-them/
Mind UK (2021). *Racism and mental health.* https://www.mind.org.uk/information-support/tips-for-everyday-living/racism-and-mental-health/
Mitchell-Miland, C., Switzer, G., White, G., Fine, M., Hollis, L., Gary-Webb, T., Morone, N., Murrell, A. and Rubio, D. (2023). 88 assessing perceptions of institutional inclusivity on burnout, intent to continue training, and perceived stress among underrepresented postdoctoral fellows and early career faculty. *Journal of Clinical and Translational Science, 7*(Suppl 1), 24. doi: 10.1017/cts.2023.171.
National Commission to Address Racism in Nursing. (2021). *Our racial reckoning statement.* American Association of Nursing. https://www.nursingworld.org/practice-policy/workforce/racism-in-nursing/RacialReckoningStatement/
Nguyen, A.N. (2025). *An Instagram post by Amanda Nguyễn 28 April 2025.* https://www.instagram.com/p/DJALY2RJ2-T/
Nwankpa, U. (2025). *The RICHER Model: Re-indigenizing wellness through evidence-based healing arts.* [Accessed 26 June 2025]. Available at: https://theuzo.com/artist-portfolio/
Olden, H.A. and Yada, F.N. (2025). Where are all the Black midwives? *Journal of Obstetric, Gynecologic, and Neonatal Nursing, 54*(3), 334–337. doi: 10.1016/j.jogn.2025.03.004.
Pollitt, P. (2016). Nurses in the Civil Rights Movement. *American Journal of Nursing, 116*(6), 50–57. doi: 10.1097/01.NAJ.0000484231.55116.8e.
Robert Wood Johnson Foundation. (2023). *Insights into nurses' experience of racism and discrimination.* https://www.statnews.com/wp-content/uploads/2023/05/rwjf473632.pdf
Robert Wood Johnson Foundation. (2025). *Leadership for better health: Building a healthy leadership across the nation.* https://www.rwjf.org/en/our-vision/focus-areas/leadership-for-better-health.html
Saad, L. (2025). *Americans' ratings of U.S. professions stay historically low. Nurses still easily top list of 23 occupations.* https://news.gallup.com/poll/655106/americans-ratings-professions-stay-historically-low.aspx
Scott, K.A., Britton, L. and McLemore, M.R. (2019). The ethics of perinatal care for Black women: Dismantling the structural racism in "Mother Blame" narratives. *The Journal of Perinatal & Neonatal Nursing, 33*(2), 108–115. doi: 10.1097/jpn.0000000000000394
Smith, C.A., Williams, E.L., Wadud, I.A. and Pirtle, W.N.L. (2021). Cite Black Women: A Critical Praxis (A Statement). *Feminist Anthropology, 2*(1), 10–17. doi: 10.1002/fea2.12040.
Solomon, D., Maxwell, C. and Castro, A. (2019). *Systematic inequality and American democracy.* https://www.americanprogress.org/issues/race/reports/2019/08/07/473003/systematic-inequality-american-democracy/
United Nations. (1948). *The Universal Declaration of Human Rights* (UDHR). United Nations General Assembly 217 A. https://docs.un.org/en/A/RES/217(III)
United Nations. (2021). *Universal Declaration of Human Rights.* https://www.un.org/sites/un2.un.org/files/2021/03/udhr.pdf (Originally published 1948).

Vo, T. (2021). Cultural alienation: A concept analysis. *Nursing Forum*, *56*(1), 160–171. doi: 10.1111/nuf.12512.
Waite, R., Beard, K. and Alexander, R. (2024). Anti-Black racism and nursing leadership. *Nurse Leader*, *22*(2), 140–145. doi: 10.1016/j.mnl.2023.12.002.
Wakefield, M.K., Williams, D.R., Le Menestrel, S. and Flaubert, J.L. and National Academies of Sciences, Engineering, and Medicine. (2021). *The future of nursing 2020-2030: Charting a path to achieve health equity*. The National Academies Press.
Walsh, H., Theeke, L.A., Ricciardi, R., Ackerman-Barger, K., Inouye, A.J., Cox, C.W. and McNelis, A.M. (2025). Racial microaggressions in nursing: "We have a long way to go". *Nursing Outlook*, *73*(2), 102347. doi: 10.1016/j.outlook.2024.102347.
Williams, D.R., Yu, Y., Jackson, J.S. and Anderson, N.B. (1997). Racial differences in physical and mental health: socioeconomic status, stress, and discrimination. *Journal of Health Psychology*, *2*(3), 335–351. doi: 10.1177/135910539700200305.
Yalom, I.D. (1970). *The theory and practice of group psychotherapy*. Basic Books.

CONCLUSION

From Rhetoric to Reality – Sustaining Anti-Racism in Nursing and Midwifery

Linda Deravin, Adrienne Lipscomb, and Hayley Mongta

Introduction

Racism remains a pervasive and deeply entrenched issue within nursing and midwifery, shaping not only the experiences of patients and practitioners but also the structures, policies and education systems that govern these professions. Despite growing awareness and inclusion efforts, systemic inequities continue to disadvantage racially minoritised groups. In this final chapter we will revisit the historical, institutional and interpersonal dimensions of racism in nursing and midwifery which have been explored in previous chapters drawing on global perspectives. If the goal is to eliminate racism from nursing and midwifery what will the future of these professions need to achieve and what might the future look like. Through a synthesis of scholarship and practice-based insights, this chapter summarises the support needed for transformation of nursing and midwifery into truly equitable, justice-based and inclusive professions where racism is called out, addressed and disrupted towards elimination.

Synthesis of Key Repeating Themes

Racism in healthcare is a multifaceted manifesting across individual, interpersonal, institutional and systemic levels (World Health Organization, 2022). In nursing and midwifery, these forms of racism are deeply embedded in professional structures, policies and everyday practices (Burnett et al., 2020; Sherwood et al., 2021; Power et al., 2021). Understanding and addressing these layers is essential for creating equitable, inclusive, justice-based and culturally safe care and work environments. Yet the challenge remains in creating these environments when structural and historical practices are so entrenched that change is often met with resistance, denial or apathy, put in the 'too hard' to implement box.

DOI: 10.4324/9781003565369-13

The roots of racism in nursing and midwifery trace back to colonial ideologies that shaped the professions' development. As Brooks and Nuku (2020) argue, colonial systems imposed Western medical models that devalued Indigenous knowledge and entrenched racialised hierarchies. These legacies continue to influence professional norms, education and leadership structures. In countries such as UK, Australia, New Zealand, Canada, Nigeria, Ghana and Sierra Leone, colonial histories have left lasting impacts on healthcare systems, contributing to workforce shortages and limiting career progression, migration and inequitable access to care. Racism also affects marginalised communities such as Gypsy, Roma and Traveller (GRT) populations, who face systemic exclusion and poor health outcomes. Anti-racist practice in these contexts requires culturally safe, relationship-based care and genuine engagement through co-design, and allyship that is partnership collaborations to flatten the hierarchical power dynamics.

Anti-racist nursing and midwifery efforts are emerging globally. In Brazil, the National Policy for the Health of the Black Population and the activism of Black nurses and midwives are advancing racial justice and culturally grounded care. In Wales, the national framework Anti-Racist Wales Action Plan is driving professional and organisational change through collaboration, co-production and accountability. In Australia, addressing racism in nursing and midwifery involves truth-telling, historical awareness and systemic reform (Sherwood et al., 2021; Strickland et al., 2023). This includes embedding cultural safety in education, regulation, and not solely service provision and delivery, and supporting Indigenous leadership in health.

Racism significantly affects midwifery and nursing outcomes, particularly for Black, Indigenous and racially minoritised populations (Niles & Drew, 2020; Shead, 2022; Bonaparte, 2023). Persistent disparities in maternal health are due to access to culturally relevant care, and representation in the workforce. Although, representation alone is not enough without embedding anti-racism strategies. In Australia, Aboriginal and Torres Strait Islander peoples face systemic barriers in both receiving care and participating in the health workforce. Advocacy from organisations like the Congress of Aboriginal and Torres Strait Islander Nurses and Midwives (CATSINaM) and the National Aboriginal Community Controlled Health Organisation (NACCHO), alongside national initiatives such as Closing the Gap (Department of Prime Minister and Cabinet, 2020) and professional accreditation and registration authorities' anti-racism policies, aim to address these inequities. Yet one country alone cannot hold back the tide of racism that permeates in many societies. It needs to be a coordinated collaborating global action for anti-racism change.

Anti-racism involves healing. Nurses and midwives engaged in justice work must address the emotional, psychological and physical toll of the real embodied consequences of racism. Healing is liberatory practice, being both for resistance and restoration, enabling individuals and communities to sustain their commitment to equity and justice. Education is a critical site for anti-racism transformation, a place for justice to start to embed in the graduating futures of the professions. Nurse educators must move beyond passive awareness to active anti-racist praxis in student recruitment, teaching, assessment and policy (Burnett et al., 2020). This must include embedding anti-racism into curricula design and delivery through justice-based methods, challenging the hidden curriculum of racial exclusion and ensuring culturally safe clinical placements. Practice education must acknowledge systemic racism and its impact on student learning and outcomes, and professional identity. Sustainable change requires personal reflexivity, institutional accountability and collective commitment (Kishimoto, 2018). Anti-racism is not a one-time initiative but an ongoing journey that demands continuous evaluation and measurable impact on workforce culture and patient outcomes (Playfair et al., 2023).

Anti-racist leadership is essential for transforming nursing and midwifery. It requires recognising the intersections of whiteness, racism, power and privilege, and actively working to dismantle inequitable structures. Representation alone is insufficient; systemic inequalities and inequities persist despite inclusion efforts, particularly in institutions like the NHS, because the leadership is replaying the status quo in many guises. Leaders from the Global Majority often face precarious positions, limiting their ability to challenge racism due to the risk to their careers. Institutional racism is perpetuated through leadership, organisational boards, policies, practices and cultural norms that uphold colonial dominance. Silence and denial of whiteness further entrench the status quo. Therefore, anti-racism must be embraced as a professional, moral and ethical imperative (Davis et al., 2024), aligning with the core values of nursing and midwifery.

So, what do we need to effectively address racism within the nursing and midwifery professions. In the next section we will examine what is needed to support anti-racism change.

Critical Conscious Reflections

For anti-racism to be sustained in nursing and midwifery, racism must be explicitly recognised as structural and systemic, not merely notional, interpersonal or attitudinal (McGibbon et al., 2014; Thorne, 2017; World Health Organization, 2022). Across Chapters 1–12, racism is consistently shown to be embedded within professional histories, education systems, regulatory frameworks, leadership cultures and clinical environments (Brooks & Nuku, 2020; Strickland et al., 2023). Without shared acknowledgement of this structural reality, institutional responses risk remaining superficial, symbolic or performative (Sue et al., 2007).

Education systems must be actively redesigned to disrupt and dismantle racism rather than merely raise awareness of it. Nursing and midwifery education often foregrounds Eurocentric knowledge systems and epistemologies marginalising Indigenous and Afrocentric knowledges, reinforcing racialised hierarchies within nursing and midwifery (McGibbon et al., 2014; Brooks & Nuku, 2020; Bourque Bearskin, 2023). This dominance perpetuates cultural isolation and identity strain among students from minoritised groups (Cook, 2024). Meaning that they don't feel belonging, supporting evidence shows that structural and interpersonal barriers undermine confidence, wellbeing and academic outcomes for these students (Caffrey et al., 2023; Pryce-Miller et al., 2023; Walker et al., 2024). The integration of critical race-informed pedagogy, and the creation of culturally safe learning and placement environments that protect racially marginalised students from harm (McGibbon et al., 2014; Kishimoto, 2018; Caffrey et al., 2023; Pryce-Miller et al., 2023; Walker et al., 2024). Practice education must move from passive equality to active anti-racism through equitable supervision, justice-based assessment and transparent reporting mechanisms for racism (Cook, 2024).

Healthcare institutions and professional organisations often maintain discriminatory policies and practices that hinder equity because those with power do not want to let go of the privilege and benefits of the system as it is in its current state. Racism is not limited to interpersonal interactions; it is embedded in governance structures, accreditation processes and workforce planning. Limited access to leadership roles, mentorship and career progression for racially minoritised nurses and midwives exemplifies structural discrimination (Sue et al., 2007). These inequities persist despite racially minoritised nurses having many relevant qualifications, publications and experiences, due to systemic racism created barriers to advancement. What is necessary is consistent truth-telling about the professions' past and the re-centring of racially minoritised marginalised voices as legitimate sources of professional and community-based knowledges (Strickland et al., 2023).

Furthermore, the ideology of colour-blindness of treating everyone 'equally', this notion denies racism and human differences let alone the lived realities of racism, preventing meaningful engagement to change and be the change that is urgently necessary (McGibbon et al., 2014; Thorne, 2017; Sherwood et al., 2021). The benchmark of how and whom equal is measured against is the colonial yardstick. That is, you are a valid human if you are White, male, Christian, English speaking, affluent, own land and property, educated, able-bodied, heterosexual, light-skinned, married and more. Anyone who doesn't measure up to the yardstick is a lesser human (Mpofu & Steyn, 2021). Denial of differences fosters resistance to anti-racism initiatives and silences critical conversations about the axes of oppressions with whiteness, racism, privilege and power. Everyday persistent behaviours, such as microaggressions, undermine racially minoritised nurses and midwives' professional identity, reinforcing exclusion and othering. These experiences accumulate over time, contributing to emotional fatigue and burnout among nurses and midwives of colour. White tears, silence and inaction further exacerbate these dynamics, to embolden some to resist engaging in difficult conversations and hard actionable anti-racism change.

For sustained anti-racism approach, organisations that include nursing and midwifery must demonstrate that healing and workforce wellbeing are essential and foundational, it is important to recognise the cumulative emotional, psychological and professional toll of racism everyday. If racism is not dealt with, it places racially minoritised practitioners at heightened risk of burnout, isolation and attrition (Sue et al., 2007; Walker, 2024; Pryce-Miller et al., 2023). Investment in healing, mentorship and workforce wellbeing is required to sustain anti-racist practice. Structured mentoring programs such as the Deadly Aboriginal and Torres Strait Islander Nursing and Midwifery Mentoring (DANMM) programme demonstrate the value of culturally anchored professional support in strengthening belonging, retention and leadership pathways (Biles et al., 2024). Institutions must also embed collective healing spaces, reflective practices and restorative responses to racial harm to prevent retraumatisation (Sue et al., 2007; Cook, 2024). Anti-racism cannot depend on the continual labour of those most harmed by racism. Instead, systems must proactively create psychologically safe environments that uphold dignity, foster belonging for all and focussed on wellbeing (Cook, 2024).

Future Directions

The pursuit of anti-racism transformation in nursing and midwifery is both urgent and complex. These professions operate within systems that have historically been shaped by colonialism, whiteness and significant structural inequities. While there is growing recognition of the need for change, progress is often slow, uneven and regularly hindered by deeply embedded barriers. At the same time, significant enablers provide valuable opportunities to disrupt or dismantle racism and build inclusive, culturally safe environments that have been shown to not only to improve the health of Black, Indigenous and racially minoritised populations but also optimise workforce development and retention, and organisational performance (McKinsey & Company, 2023; Biles et al., 2024). Understanding these complex dynamics is essential for shaping meaningful and sustainable transformative reform and promoting and supporting the following enablers is critical to success.

Institutional accountability is another non-negotiable condition for change. Anti-racism cannot be sustained through goodwill alone; it must be embedded within governance, accreditation, performance frameworks and regulatory oversight metrics (Burnett et al., 2020; Davis et al., 2024). Where accountability mechanisms are absent or inconsistently applied, racism persists through organisational silence, denial or inaction (Sue et al., 2007; Thorne, 2017). Sustainable anti-racism also requires the redistribution of power. Racially minoritised and marginalised nurses, midwives, students and communities must not only be consulted but must hold genuine agency and authority in collaborative decision-making, curriculum governance, policy design and research leadership (Kishimoto, 2018; Strickland et al., 2023; Biles et al., 2024). Without this structural shift, institutions risk reproducing tokenism and dominant whiteness pull of the system, rather than anti-racism transformation.

Acknowledging the contributions of Black, Indigenous and Global South nurses and midwives is foundational for reconstructing culturally responsive professional identity and unlearning and disrupting Eurocentric dominance. Truth-telling initiatives challenge dominant narratives and create space for inclusive and accurate learning and embedding of history. This recognition fosters belonging and validates the expertise of racially minoritised practitioners and communities. Creating such spaces for racially minoritised nurses and midwives to share lived experiences disrupts the dominant white Eurocentric narratives and informs anti-racism strategies (Gillborn, 2024; Parkin & Johnson, 2024). Counter-storytelling foregrounds systemic critique and ensures that reform efforts are grounded in the realities of those most affected by racism.

Leadership and governance reform is essential. Senior leaders, boards and regulators must be held accountable for measurable anti-racism outcomes tied to their performance review, salary and bonuses and organisational evaluation (Strickland et al., 2023; Davis et al., 2024). Leadership is central to cultural change, anti-racist leadership in nursing and midwifery involves recognising the intersection of racism, power and privilege, and actively working to transform institutions from within to create equitable liberatory environments. Enhancing Black, Brown and Indigenous representation in leadership and supervisory roles signals a commitment to equity. Mentoring programs, such as the Deadly Aboriginal and Torres Strait Islander Nursing and Midwifery Mentoring (DANMM) initiative (Biles et al., 2024), strengthen professional development and belonging. Representation alone is insufficient; leadership structures must be transformed so that racially marginalised leaders are supported, protected and empowered to drive institutional change and lift others in their communities up in the organisation, e.g., through mentoring (Sue et al., 2007; Biles et al., 2024).

These efforts dismantle barriers to promotion and create environments where diversity is integral rather than exceptional. Organisational willingness to reform discriminatory structures, revise policies and embed equity into accreditation processes creates supportive conditions for systemic transformation (Burnett et al., 2020).

Integrating anti-racism frameworks into nursing and midwifery curricula empowers practitioners to challenge discrimination. The inclusion of Black, Global South and Indigenous history, health and culture, taught with a strengths-based position can assist with the decolonising of health curricula, ensuring that nurses and midwives understand the impact of coloniality (Moloney & Stuart, 2025). Culturally responsive pedagogies, safe open spaces for dialogue, we should not need to be brave to speak up and out, it should just be that way to share a diversity of innovation and creativity, and strategies that cultivate critical consciousness are essential for disrupting systemic inequities.

Partnerships with communities, such as GRT representatives, enhance program design and delivery. Collaborative approaches with minoritised and marginalised communities ensure that cultural strengths and knowledges are recognised rather than marginalised because it is seen as lesser in necessity. Global solidarity movements and grassroots activism further reinforce local efforts, connecting anti-racism work to broader social justice agendas (Davis et al., 2024). Relational models built on respect, reciprocity and genuine listening underpin culturally safe care. These approaches prioritise fairness, inclusion and wellbeing for both staff and service users. Evidence-based models of culturally safe practice provide practical guidance for embedding these principles into everyday care.

Institutional commitment is equally critical. Measurable anti-racism outcomes, transparent mechanisms for tracking progress and cross-sector collaboration provide the structural enablers for lasting change. Continuous professional development that emphasises cultural humility helps embed anti-racist principles into practice which can be sustained over time.

Despite the many enablers outlined, there are also significant barriers to change present in nursing and midwifery. One of the most enduring barriers is the exclusion of Black, Brown and Indigenous contributions from professional histories as this erasure reinforces systemic bias and perpetuates a narrow and Eurocentric narrative (Bourque-Bearskin, 2023). Without recognition of diverse role models, students and practitioners from minoritised and marginalised backgrounds experience diminished visibility, belonging and agency. This is not a new concept, 'You can't be what you can't see' has been identified as a barrier in many areas, from higher education to elite sports (Kinnane et al., 2014; Stronach et al., 2023).

Call to Action

Even when anti-racism policies exist, implementation is often inconsistent. Leadership accountability is weak, and resources to support transformative reform are limited. This results in tokenistic and/or performative gestures rather than transformative actions. Difficulty in disrupting established stubborn hierarchies and privilege sustains institutional inertia, slowing progress towards equity.

The path towards anti-racism nursing and midwifery requires more than policy rhetoric; it demands structural transformation, cultural humility and sustained accountability. Future efforts must prioritise:

- Embedding anti-racism into accreditation, curricula design and professional standards.
- Strengthening leadership accountability through measurable equity outcomes.
- Amplifying and integrating minoritised and marginalised voices in research, education and policy.
- Investing in academic anti-racism development and culturally safe pedagogical strategies.
- Proactively supporting wellbeing among racially minoritised practitioners to mitigate racialised trauma and burnout.

Advancing anti-racism in nursing and midwifery requires both global solidarity and sustained local commitment. As evidenced across Wales, Brazil, Nigeria, Australia and the GRT community context, international knowledge-sharing strengthens accountability, deepens political will and prevents the isolation of anti-racism work within individual institutions or nations (Gillborn, 2024; Parkin & Johnson, 2024; Strickland et al., 2023). Yet solidarity alone is insufficient without long-term resourcing and structural support. Anti-racism must be adequately funded, institutionally prioritised and embedded through sustained investment in education reform, leadership development, community partnership and cultural safety infrastructure (Burnett et al., 2020; Davis et al., 2024; Biles et al., 2024).

Ultimately, anti-racism change is not a peripheral special interest project, it is central to ethical, equitable and culturally safe care. By leveraging enablers and disrupting or dismantling the persistent barriers from systemic racism, nursing and midwifery can move towards a future where diversity is celebrated, justice is embedded and health systems serve all communities with dignity and respect. To move from rhetoric to reality, anti-racism must be embedded as core business across nursing and midwifery education, practice, leadership and regulation. Accreditation standards, professional codes and regulatory frameworks must explicitly require demonstrable anti-racist knowledge, skills, behaviours and metrics for accountability, rather than treating anti-racism as an optional 'nice to have' initiative or professional attribute (Burnett et al., 2020; Strickland et al., 2023; Davis et al., 2024).

Closing Thoughts

The journey towards anti-racism in nursing and midwifery is not a single act or isolated occurrence, it is a lifelong process of learning, reflection and transformation. It calls on every individual whether they be a practitioner, educator or leader to move beyond passive awareness to actively embracing the responsibility for dismantling inequities and disrupting ambivalence and naivety to challenge racism in all its forms. Anti-racism in nursing and midwifery is a transformative process that demands historical reckoning, systemic critique and courageous leadership. It calls for a shift from individual bias to institutional accountability, from representation to structural change and from passive inclusion to actively implementing justice-based practice.

By foundationally embedding anti-racism into education, practice and policy, health professions can move towards a more equitable and liberatory future. When individuals and institutions commit to this lifelong process they create continuous ripples of change that go beyond the workplace to strengthen and uplift communities, and build a legacy of fairness for generations to come for all. Stand up, act, unsettle the status quo and do anti-racism change. Over to you.

Reflective Activity

Having read the chapter, we invite you to reflect on your key learning and its implications for your professional practice as a nurse or midwife using Bain et al.'s (2002) 5R framework (pp. 13–15):

- Reporting – What is it in your situation you want to transform after reading this chapter?

- Responding – What are your personal observations regarding your own situation/context in relation to what is raised in this chapter?
- Relating – What is/are the theoretical/research/data/legislative, etc., understandings relationship to under consideration in this chapter that you could apply to your situation/context?
- Reasoning – Identify how the chapter findings matter to your situation/context and how will you interrogate your situation/context and what will help you from this chapter?
- Reconstructing – Identify your action plans to reframe and rebuild a transformative way forward to change from the situation in your context.

References

Biles, B., Christian, B., Marshall, C., McMillan, F., Sara, G., Anderson, J., Davies, N., Fealy, S. and Biles, J. (2024). 'DANMM that's good!': Evaluating the feasibility and acceptability of the Deadly Aboriginal and Torres Strait Islander Nursing and Midwifery Mentoring (DANMM) Programme across rural, regional and metropolitan NSW—A collaborative study protocol. *BMJ Open*, 14, e079416.

Bonaparte, A.D. (2023). Regulating childbirth: Physicians and granny midwives in South Carolina. In J.C. Oparah and A.D. Bonaparte (eds.) *Birthing Justice: Black Women, Pregnancy and Childbirth*. Routledge (pp. 6–18).

Bourque Bearskin, M.L. (2023). Decolonization the what, why and how: A treaties on Indigenous nursing knowledge. *Nursing Philosophy*, 24, e12430-n/a.

Brooks, G. and Nuku, K. (2020). Why we aren't celebrating Florence's birthday. *Kai Tiaki Nursing New Zealand*, 26, 34–35.

Burnett, A., Moorley, C., Grant, J., Kahin, M., Sagoo, R., Rivers, E., Deravin, L. and Darbyshire, P. (2020). Dismantling racism in education: In 2020, the year of the nurse & midwife, "it's time." *Nurse Educ Today*, 93, 104532.

Cook, F. (2024). Representation and sense of belonging for people of the Global Majority in higher education. *Student Engagement in Higher Education Journal*, 5, 111–128.

Davis, S., Martin-Holland, J., Gemeda, M.L. and Mitchell, D.A. (2024). An anti-racism framework for educating nursing professionals. *Nursing Outlook*, 72, 102242.

Department of Prime Minister and Cabinet. (2020). *National Agreement on Closing the Gap* [Online]. Commonwealth of Australia. https://www.closingthegap.gov.au/national-agreement/national-agreement-closing-the-gap

Gillborn, D. (2024). *White Lies: Racism, Education and Critical Race Theory*. Routledge.

Kinnane, S., Wilks, J.L., Wilson, K., Hughes, T. and Thomas, S. (2014). *'Can't Be What You Can't See': The Transition of Aboriginal and Torres Strait Islander Students into Higher Education; Final Report 2014*. University of Notre Dame Australia; Southern Cross University.

Kishimoto, K. (2018). Anti-racist pedagogy: From faculty's self-reflection to organizing within and beyond the classroom. *Race Ethnicity and Education*, 21, 540–554.

McGibbon, E., Mulaudzi, F.M., Didham, P., Barton, S. and Sochan, A. (2014). Toward decolonizing nursing: The colonization of nursing and strategies for increasing the counter-narrative. *Nursing Inquiry*, 21, 179–191.

McKinsey and Company. (2023). *Diversity matters even more: The case for holistic impact*. https://www.mckinsey.com/featured-insights/diversity-and-inclusion/diversity-matters-even-more-the-case-for-holistic-impact#/

Moloney, A. and Stuart, L. (2025). Cultural safety and clinical safety: A symbiotic relationship for improving Aboriginal and Torres Strait Islander Peoples and Communities' health outcomes. *Contemporary Nurse: A Journal for the Australian Nursing Profession*, 1–11. https://doi.org/10.1080/10376178.2025.2573155

Mpofu, W. and Steyn, M. (2021). The trouble with the human. In M. Steyn and W. Mpofu (eds.), *Decolonisng the Human: Reflections from Africa on Difference and Oppression.* Wits University Press (pp. 1–24).

Niles, P.M. and Drew, M. (2020). *Constructing the Modern Amer* [Online]. https://nursingclio.org/2020/10/22/constructing-the-modern-american-midwife-white-supremacy-and-white-feminism-collide/

Playfair, C., Hunt, G. and Dacosta, C. (2023). Developing anti-racist undergraduate nursing education: Themes and action. *British Journal of Nursing*, 32, 746–751.

Power, T., Geia, L., Adams, K., Drummond, A., Saunders, V., Stuart, L., Deravin, L., Tuala, M., Roe, Y., Sherwood, J., Rowe Minniss, F. and West, R. (2021). Beyond 2020: Addressing racism through transformative Indigenous health and cultural safety education. *Journal of Clinical Nursing*, 30, e32–e35.

Pryce-Miller, M., Bliss, E., Airey, A., Garvey, A. and Pennington, C.R. (2023). The lived experiences of racial bias for Black, Asian and minority ethnic students in practice: A hermeneutic phenomenological study. *Nurse Education in Practice*, 66, 103532.

Shead, S. (2022). "Granny" midwife to nurse-midwife: The decline of Southern Black midwifery in the 20th century. *Historical Perspectives: Santa Clara University Undergraduate Journal of History, Series II*, 27, 9.

Sherwood, J., West, R., Geia, L., Drummond, A., Power, T., Stuart, L. and Deravin, L. 2021. "Taking our blindfolds off": Acknowledging the vision of First Nations peoples for nursing and midwifery. *Australian Journal of Advanced Nursing*, 38, 1–5.

Strickland, K., Deravin, L., Williamson, M., Atherfold, C., West, C., Nightingale, K. and Bonner, A. (2023). An apology to Aboriginal and Torres Islander people: A moment of truth for the nursing and midwifery professions. *Collegian*, 30, 207–209.

Stronach, M., O'Shea, M. and Maxwell, H. (2023). 'You can't be what you can't see': Indigenous Australian sportswomen as powerful role models. *Sport in Society*, 26, 970–984.

Sue, D.W., Capodilupo, C.M., Torino, G.C., Bucceri, J.M., Holder, A.M.B., Nadal, K.L. and Esqulin, M. (2007). Racial microaggression in everyday life: Implications for clinical practice. *American Psychologist*, 62, 271–286.

Thorne, S. (2017). Isn't it high time we talked openly about racism? *Nursing Inquiry*, *24*, e12219. https://doi.org/10.1111/nin.12219

Walker, C.R., Gunasinghe, C., Harwood, H., Ehsan, A., Ahmed, F., Dorrington, S. and Rhead, R.D. (2024). Ethnic inequalities during clinical placement: A qualitative study of student nurses' experiences within the London National Health Service. *Journal of Advanced Nursing*, 80, 1497–1510.

World Health Organization. (2022). *Strengthening Primary Health Care to Tackle Racial Discrimination, Promote Intercultural Services and Reduce Health Inequities. Research Brief* [Online]. World Health Organization. https://www.who.int/publications/i/item/9789240057104

INDEX